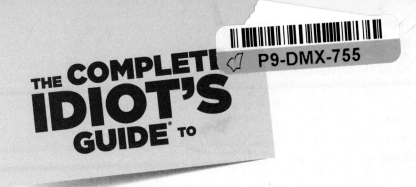

THE COMPLETE IDIOT'S GUIDE® TO

The Mediterranean Diet

by Kimberly A. Tessmer, RD, LD, and Chef Stephanie Green, RD

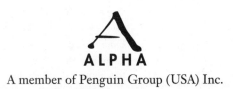

ALPHA

A member of Penguin Group (USA) Inc.

ALPHA BOOKS

Published by the Penguin Group

Penguin Group (USA) Inc., 375 Hudson Street, New York, New York 10014, USA

Penguin Group (Canada), 90 Eglinton Avenue East, Suite 700, Toronto, Ontario M4P 2Y3, Canada (a division of Pearson Penguin Canada Inc.)

Penguin Books Ltd., 80 Strand, London WC2R 0RL, England

Penguin Ireland, 25 St. Stephen's Green, Dublin 2, Ireland (a division of Penguin Books Ltd.)

Penguin Group (Australia), 250 Camberwell Road, Camberwell, Victoria 3124, Australia (a division of Pearson Australia Group Pty. Ltd.)

Penguin Books India Pvt. Ltd., 11 Community Centre, Panchsheel Park, New Delhi—110 017, India

Penguin Group (NZ), 67 Apollo Drive, Rosedale, North Shore, Auckland 1311, New Zealand (a division of Pearson New Zealand Ltd.)

Penguin Books (South Africa) (Pty.) Ltd., 24 Sturdee Avenue, Rosebank, Johannesburg 2196, South Africa

Penguin Books Ltd., Registered Offices: 80 Strand, London WC2R 0RL, England

International Standard Book Number: 978-1-61564-046-1
Library of Congress Catalog Card Number: 2010906822

12 11 10   8 7 6 5 4 3 2 1

Interpretation of the printing code: The rightmost number of the first series of numbers is the year of the book's printing; the rightmost number of the second series of numbers is the number of the book's printing. For example, a printing code of 10-1 shows that the first printing occurred in 2010.

Printed in the United States of America

Note: This publication contains the opinions and ideas of its authors. It is intended to provide helpful and informative material on the subject matter covered. It is sold with the understanding that the authors and publisher are not engaged in rendering professional services in the book. This book should not be construed as medical advice, nor should it take the place of regularly scheduled appointments with your physician or treatment that your physician has prescribed. If the reader requires personal assistance or advice, a competent professional should be consulted. Please consult with your health-care provider for medical advice and before starting any type of new eating plan.

The authors and publisher specifically disclaim any responsibility for any liability, loss, or risk, personal or otherwise, which is incurred as a consequence, directly or indirectly, of the use and application of any of the contents of this book.

Most Alpha books are available at special quantity discounts for bulk purchases for sales promotions, premiums, fund-raising, or educational use. Special books, or book excerpts, can also be created to fit specific needs.

For details, write: Special Markets, Alpha Books, 375 Hudson Street, New York, NY 10014.

Publisher: *Marie Butler-Knight*

Associate Publisher: *Mike Sanders*

Senior Managing Editor: *Billy Fields*

Senior Acquisitions Editor: *Paul Dinas*

Development Editor: *Lynn Northrup*

Senior Production Editor: *Janette Lynn*

Copy Editor: *Jaime Julian Wagner*

Cover Designer: *William Thomas*

Book Designers: *William Thomas, Rebecca Batchelor*

Indexer: *Angie Bess*

Layout: *Ayanna Lacey*

Proofreader: *Laura Caddell*

Contents

Appendixes

Introduction

Have you been curious about trying the Mediterranean diet but not quite sure where to start? Do you want to skip all of the scientific mumbo jumbo and get right to the heart of the matter? Then this book should be your starting point. It will help to spell out all aspects of this ever-popular heart-healthy diet in terms everyone will understand. It is full of practical information, tips, and advice. And let's not forget the mouthwatering recipes and corresponding meal plans that will help get you started immediately.

After reading this book, you will come away with not just an understanding of what the Mediterranean diet is all about and how to follow it, but also with a much stronger understanding of good nutrition and how it is related to your health. This book was written for the person who wants to live a longer and healthier life—and we would guess that's most of us. If you are ready to make changes and take control of your life and your health, then this is the book for you!

How We've Organized This Book

To help make this book easy to follow and use, we have divided the chapters into four different parts. Each part brings its own unique information to the book and helps guide you easily through the vast information that surrounds the Mediterranean diet.

Part 1, Eating the Mediterranean Way, gets right into the background of the Mediterranean diet and what makes it Mediterranean. We explore all of the health benefits that this diet has to offer. There is something for everyone to relate to, whether you already have health issues or you just want to lower your risk for health issues. You get the inside scoop on all the food groups that make up the Mediterranean Diet Pyramid along with their Mediterranean guidelines. The Mediterranean diet isn't just a "diet." You discover all aspects important to this style of eating from food to lifestyle.

Part 2, The Basics of the Mediterranean Diet, provides you with the tools and knowledge you need to make this diet your own. We show you how the Mediterranean diet stacks up against other popular diets you may have tried, have thought of trying, or have heard of. If you are considering using this diet not only for good health but to lose a few extra pounds, this part spells out the strategies you need to be successful. Helpful tips get you started in transitioning your current diet to more of a Mediterranean style. We take a comprehensive look at all of the foods and beverages associated with the Mediterranean diet, including olive oil, whole grains, fruits, vegetables, fish, seafood, nuts, seeds, legumes, meats, eggs, dairy products, and red wine.

Part 3, Treasures of the Mediterranean Diet, provides you with the knowledge to understand what is in the foods of the Mediterranean that make them so health-promoting. This part examines the facts on the macronutrients, including fats, carbohydrates, and protein; it also takes a look at fiber. You become very familiar with the micronutrients including vitamins, minerals, antioxidants, and phytonutrients—all the nutrients you knew were healthy but weren't quite sure why. This part answers your questions and helps you to make the food and nutrition connection and how it all relates back to the health benefits of the Mediterranean diet.

Part 4, Savor the Flavors of the Mediterranean, starts out by exploring the many herbs and spices associated with the Mediterranean that add not only their unique flavor but also health benefits to your foods. We include fabulous and tasty recipes that incorporate many of the foods, beverages, herbs, and spices we discuss in the book. These recipes help bring it all together, giving you the ability to create healthy dishes that incorporate Mediterranean health benefits. We then use these recipes to create four weeks of seasonal meal plans that will aid you in starting this amazing diet immediately and making it part of your everyday life.

Extras

As you read through the book, you will notice bonus boxes that contain definitions, tips, warnings, and miscellaneous information to help in your understanding of the subject matter.

DEFINITION

These boxes provide you with definitions that are relevant to the topic at hand.

TO YOUR HEALTH

Check these boxes for tips that impact your health on everything from foods to the nutrients they contain.

GOOD TO KNOW

These boxes contain warnings you should keep in mind when it comes to foods or your health.

HEALTHY MORSELS

These boxes are full of tidbits of information that might just be a surprise to you.

Acknowledgments

From Kimberly:

I want to extend a special thank you to my co-author Stephanie Green, RD, who worked so diligently with me to pull this book together. Thank you for all of your long, hard work and expertise! It was a complete pleasure to work with you.

A special thanks to my literary agent, Jessica Faust, and her crew at BookEnds, LLC, for making this project happen and for making the entire process run so smoothly.

Many thanks to people who lent their expertise: Nour El-Zibdeh, RD; Aphrodite Dikeakos, MS, RD; and Jo Ann Hattner, MPH, RD.

I am grateful to Birthe Creutz, Director of Finance and License Manager, at Oldways Preservation Trust (www.oldwayspt.org) for granting us permission to use several images in the book and for working with us to get just the right ones.

On a personal note, I want to dedicate this book to my two favorite girls. In loving memory of my beautiful and courageous Mom, Nancy Bradford, who always taught and showed me that all things are possible and passed on to me her incredible passion for helping others. And to my wonderful little girl, Tori, who was so patient as I wrote this book and who puts a smile on my face every day. You are the light of my life. A special thank you to my wonderful husband, Greg, for his endless love, support, and encouragement. I couldn't have taken the time to write this book without you! Thank you to my Dad, Don Bradford, and my sister, Sheryl Brodsky, for their constant love, support, and encouragement. A heartfelt thank you to my incredible extended family, my sister-in-law, Lori Milloy, and my in-laws, Fred and Lois Tessmer. Thank you for all the babysitting as well as your love and support. A big thank you to *all* my friends and family!

From Stephanie:

Much appreciation and thanks to my co-author Kimberly Tessmer, RD, LD, for holding my hand during the process of this book and offering guidance and support.

Big heartfelt thanks to all of my assistants who worked alongside me on the recipes and shopped, chopped, washed, and ate! Joanna Burnett, Linnea Caldeen, Joey Morgan, Lindsay L'vova, and Elizabeth Milburn.

I want to dedicate this book to my husband, Duane, for his gracious support.

Special Thanks to the Technical Reviewer

The recipes in *The Complete Idiot's Guide to the Mediterranean Diet* were reviewed by an expert who double-checked the accuracy of what you'll learn here to help us ensure that this book gives you everything you need to know about the Mediterranean diet. Special thanks are extended to Rowann Gilman, a freelance New York City–based food magazine and cookbook editor and writer.

Trademarks

All terms mentioned in this book that are known to be or are suspected of being trademarks or service marks have been appropriately capitalized. Alpha Books and Penguin Group (USA) Inc. cannot attest to the accuracy of this information. Use of a term in this book should not be regarded as affecting the validity of any trademark or service mark.

Eating the Mediterranean Way

The first part of this book starts with the first steps you should take before beginning any type of new eating style: learning all you can about a plan's background and the components that make up the diet. If you are wondering why you should eat the Mediterranean way and how it can benefit your health, this part helps to answer those questions by explaining all of the benefits currently attributable to this way of eating—and this way of life. We explain the food groups that make up the building blocks of the Mediterranean diet and give you the inside scoop on what makes them essential to this way of eating.

What Makes It Mediterranean?

In This Chapter

- Mediterranean diet history
- What's it all about?
- Implementing this new lifestyle
- Debunking the most common myth
- What makes the Mediterranean diet unique?

The Mediterranean diet is a style of eating or an eating pattern that has been around for many years. It has stood the test of time and has pretty much come out unscathed compared to other "diets" on the market. Even though it has been around for such a long time, it is one of the least publicized diet plans around—it seems the healthiest and smartest ones always are!

Before embarking on any diet plan or new eating pattern, you should have a good understanding of its history, including what it entails and where it came from. If you are going to trust your health to a new way of life, you need to learn all you can, starting at the beginning.

A Little Background

When you think of the Mediterranean, you may conjure up thoughts of blue water, pristine coastlines, spectacular scenery, and a rich culture. However, experts see something very different in this area, and they are beginning to appreciate more and more the eating style of the people who inhabit these regions. Studies confirm that their style of eating is not only healthful for your heart but for your overall well-being.

The Mediterranean diet was actually first developed back in the 1940s but didn't gain any real recognition until the 1990s. The Mediterranean diet is known for its heart-healthy eating style and permanent way of life. Once you embrace this lifestyle, you will experience a way of eating—and living—that people throughout the Mediterranean regions have practiced for many centuries. The results will be an everyday way of living that helps you to look and feel your best.

HEALTHY MORSELS

A 2003 study in the *New England Journal of Medicine* that followed 2,000 adults concluded that adherence to the principles of the traditional Mediterranean diet is associated with a longer survival rate.

Where It Came From

There isn't just one single Mediterranean diet; in fact, there are close to 16 countries that surround this region. Diet preferences can vary depending on each country's ethnic background, religion, culture, economy, and agricultural differences. However, no matter what the slight differences are among them, the eating patterns of these countries all have a great deal in common.

For our purposes we will discuss the most common Mediterranean diet, which is based on the traditional eating style of people within the Mediterranean region such as Crete, Greece, and southern Italy. By "traditional," we refer to a time, around the 1960s, when rates of chronic diseases in these areas were among the lowest in the world and the life expectancy of adults was at its highest.

Who It Came From

Dr. Ancel Keys, an American physiologist and nutritionist who lived in Italy, developed the original idea for the Mediterranean diet and discovered the health benefits that accompany it. In 1958, he began his 20 year landmark study (popularly known as the Seven Countries Study) that analyzed the role of diet in heart disease throughout seven countries. In 1970, he published the results of this study, establishing the basis of what would eventually be known as the Mediterranean diet.

In general, the study revealed that people in these areas who followed a Mediterranean-style eating pattern had lower percentages of death due to cardiovascular disease. Dr. Keys discovered that people in these areas consumed fewer *saturated fats* and *trans fats*; more *healthy fats*, especially monounsaturated fats; less dairy; and more fruits, vegetables, nuts, legumes, and whole grains than other diets around the world. One of the strongest conclusions that came from this study was that a higher intake of saturated fat put one at risk for cardiovascular disease.

DEFINITION

Healthy fat is a term used for those fats that are unsaturated, such as mono-unsaturated, polyunsaturated, and omega-3 fatty acids. These fats help to reduce the risk for heart disease through their various functions in the body, as opposed to **saturated fats** and **trans fats,** which are unhealthful fats that do the opposite. See Chapter 14 for a further explanation of all the types of fats.

Although it was Dr. Keys who first developed the idea behind the Mediterranean diet, it was another group of professionals that introduced the concept as a whole. In 1993, the Oldways Preservation & Exchange Trust, along with the Harvard School of Public Health and the World Health Organization, first introduced the total concept of the Mediterranean diet at a conference in Cambridge, Massachusetts. The Mediterranean diet, along with the Mediterranean Diet Pyramid (which we discuss in Chapter 3), have become known worldwide as the gold standard for dietary patterns that promote heart health and long life. As time goes by, researchers are discovering even more proven effects of sticking to this diet, including healthy weight loss, a lower risk of cancer, improved cognitive function, improvement for those dealing with depression, better controlled blood sugar, and relief from inflammation.

A Healthier Approach to Eating

The irony of this diet is that the people of the Mediterranean consume more fat on the whole than what is recommended for a typical Western diet, yet they have lower mortality rates from cardiovascular disease. The reason, you ask? Simple—they eat much less saturated fats (or "bad" fats) and much more unsaturated fats (or "good" fats). Keep in mind that even though including healthier fats is key, it is not the only factor that results in lower mortality rates. It is also the many other healthful foods that make up a healthy eating pattern, as well as overall lifestyle habits, such as increased physical activity and lower stress levels, that makes this diet a healthier approach.

It is no one food but rather a combination of foods that appears to be responsible for the positive health benefits of this style of eating. In addition, people from the Mediterranean regions tend to eat slowly, use smaller plates, eat rich foods sparingly, and eat food that is in season. It's all about the diet as a whole—the way foods are prepared and the recipes that are used on a day-to-day basis that is the foundation of this healthy approach to eating.

This follows closely the position of the American Dietetic Association, which emphasizes that it is not individual foods that are key to good health but rather the total diet or overall eating pattern that is the most important focus of a healthful eating style. Many experts seem to agree on this approach.

Key Components of the Diet

The Mediterranean diet is not complicated; however, it relies on several key components to work its magic. Once you become familiar with all of the basic components of the Mediterranean diet, you can begin to set goals for yourself to slowly make necessary changes.

To make this diet a permanent part of your life, it's essential that you adapt it to your own personal lifestyle and preferences. The more components you are able to incorporate into your life, the better your body will function and the more health benefits you will reap. The more this diet becomes your own, the more successful you will be at sticking with it—and the more it will become second nature.

Key components of the Mediterranean diet include:

- Minimally processed foods.

- Lots of fruits and vegetables that are fresh and preferably locally grown.

- Whole grains such as pastas, cereals, breads, and other grain products.

- Legumes (dried beans), nuts, and seeds.

- Moderate amounts of fish and shellfish with low to moderate amounts of poultry, eggs, and other lean meats to help meet protein needs. Red meats are used very little, if at all.

- Moderate amounts of dairy products (preferably fat-free or low-fat).

- Healthy, unsaturated fats from fish, avocados, olive oil, and canola oil. Butter, margarine, and other saturated and trans fats are avoided.

- Herbs and spices to flavor foods instead of using salt.

- Sugars that come from natural sources such as fruit and honey.

- Red wine consumed in small amounts with meals (in moderation, of course).
  If you don't drink, don't start. You can always use purple grape juice as an
  alternative.

Adopting the Mediterranean Way of Life

Although a move to the Mediterranean might sound inviting, it isn't necessary to
reap the benefits of this region's healthy eating habits. You can adapt your behavior
to incorporate this way of life by gaining the proper knowledge and making smarter
food choices.

GOOD TO KNOW

Adapting to this new way of life takes time. Don't try to change everything all in
one day. Your goal should be to approach the changes step by step.

What Makes This Diet So Healthy?

As you begin to adopt this way of life, it is important for you to know exactly why
the Mediterranean diet is said to be so healthy. Many factors contribute to the health
benefits, and it has been proven in numerous studies that people of the Mediterranean
are indeed healthy.

It is the multiple factors at work that provides the health benefits of the
Mediterranean diet. It incorporates an abundance of nutritional powerhouse foods
working together that cannot be replaced by a supplement. This translates into a diet
that is rich in unprocessed foods, lean protein, essential vitamins and minerals, whole
grains, fiber, antioxidants, and healthy fats. It is the whole nutritional package and
doesn't leave out any part of a well-balanced, healthy diet. Add the other aspects of
this healthy lifestyle and you have a punch so powerful it can knock down your risk
for a slew of fatal health conditions.

Keep in mind though that a diet can only be as healthy as you allow it to be. In other
words, the more closely you follow it, the more benefits you will reap. If you decide
this diet is for you and you are counting on its health benefits, you need to ensure
you have the knowledge and the motivation to adopt this new way of life to its fullest.
Commitment is key!

HEALTHY MORSELS

A study by the *British Medical Journal* (BMJ) in September 2008 concluded that greater adherence to a Mediterranean diet is associated with a significant improvement in one's health. Proof is the decrease of overall mortality by 9 percent, death from cardiovascular diseases by 9 percent, decrease in cancer by 6 percent, and decrease in the incidence of Parkinson's disease and Alzheimer's disease by 13 percent. This and other studies concerning the Mediterranean diet help encourage people to adopt a Mediterranean-type eating style for primary prevention of major chronic health conditions. It may seem like just a bunch of numbers, but these studies are the proof you may need to answer that burning question: "Why should I change?"

Helpful Tips for Getting Started

Now that you're aware of the key components of this diet, it's time to start making some changes. However, making changes all at once can be overwhelming and often can undermine your best intentions. The most important concept is to gradually implement new changes while continuing to implement the ones you have already made. If it seems overwhelming, try writing down your goals weekly to keep track of your successes.

Here are some tips for beginning the shift to the Mediterranean diet:

- Substitute and/or replace foods slowly. You don't want to jump in all at once, especially if your diet needs a lot of help. A good way to start is to replace side dishes and then move on from there.

- Start by using olive oil and/or canola oil as your main fat source instead of unhealthy fats such as margarine or butter. Consider using it in cooking, as a replacement for your favorite salad dressing, or on bread for items such as garlic toast.

- Fill at least half of your plate with fruits and/or vegetables. Leave the rest for whole grains, lean meat, fish, or beans.

- Visit your local produce markets to buy some of your produce (or start your own garden!).

- Introduce a new fruit and/or vegetable each week to your meal plans to include variety in your diet. Don't be afraid to experience new foods.

- Substitute grilled, broiled, or steamed fish instead of red meat or other high-fat meats at least twice a week. Each week, reduce the number of meals where red meat (or other high-fat meat) is served—and decrease the portion sizes as well.

- Begin to replace refined grains (such as white bread, white rice, or white pasta) for whole grains (such as whole-wheat bread, brown rice, and whole-wheat pasta).

- Try out whole grains common to the Mediterranean such as barley, bulgur, and couscous by using some new recipes.

- Plan a few meatless meals each week—make legumes or beans the main focus of those meals.

- Switch to soft or semisoft cheeses that are low in fat (such as low-fat goat cheese or part-skim mozzarella), fat-free milk, and fat-free or low-fat plain yogurt.

- Season your foods and recipes with herbs and spices instead of salt. It may take some practice and experimentation to get good at it!

- Begin cooking more of your meals from scratch, cutting back on the amount of processed foods. Invest in a few good Mediterranean cookbooks to help get you started and get those creative juices flowing.

- Replace sweets, baked goods, and other fat- and sugar-laden desserts and treats with fresh fruit, fruit-based desserts, and/or nuts.

- Work on making mealtime a special time of the day. Eat at the table with the family, and set aside enough time to slow down and enjoy your meal.

- Accept the fact that it is okay to revert back to your traditional diet once in awhile. If you don't have control of a meal—say you're at a friend's house—then do the best you can. Don't beat yourself up.

- If it is approved by your doctor, try adding a glass of red wine at dinner. If you don't drink, try substituting purple grape juice to reap some of the benefits.

TO YOUR HEALTH

Always consult your physician before you start any type of new diet or exercise plan.

These are all simple suggestions to help get you started, but remember that you don't have to tackle them all at the same time. You will read many tips and helpful hints throughout this book that will assist you in transitioning your diet. Once you begin to incorporate some of these suggestions into your daily life, you will begin to realize how simple, healthful, and tasty this diet can be. It should become a permanent way of life!

Other Lifestyle Factors

The Mediterranean lifestyle is not only about its tasty foods and red wine (wouldn't that be nice!). You need to incorporate all of the lifestyle factors to derive all the potential health benefits. Making these types of lifestyle changes can help to change you in mind, body, and spirit.

Incorporating these types of changes means breaking a few bad habits and replacing them with good ones. How long do you let those bad habits go on before admitting to them, taking responsibility for them, and doing something about them? Is it time to quit smoking, get moving, reduce your stress, and generally take better care of yourself? There is no time like the present! And the good news is that it is never too late to get started on the Mediterranean way of life to help increase longevity and reduce risk for chronic diseases. In fact, the sooner you begin, the better chance you have to begin reversing some of the damage that may have already been done. Your efforts will be well rewarded.

Physical Activity

Although people of the Mediterranean consume plenty of healthy fats and a bit of wine with their meals, they do not seem to be plagued with weight problems. They are able to balance the amount of food they consume with regular physical activity. This is an extremely important part of what makes the Mediterranean way of life a healthy one. The key is that these people make activity part of their lifestyle, not something they have to do.

No matter how you include physical activity in your life, the answer is to just do it. Physical activity can take many forms, and it is important to choose an activity you enjoy. Being physically active needs to be a habit that you adopt for the rest of your life. Just like any other habit, it takes time, perseverance, and work to get that habit to stick. You don't have to join the nearest gym and work out for two hours a day—unless you want to, of course—but you do need to be active on a daily basis to get any type of health benefit from it.

The Dietary Guidelines for Americans stresses at least 30 minutes of moderate physical activity on most days to provide essential health benefits for adults. In addition, increasing the time or intensity of your physical activity provides even more health benefits. Walking in your neighborhood or on your lunch break at work can be a great start. You can look into dancing, yoga, walking groups, swimming, or whatever you enjoy.

The keys are to get started, do something you enjoy, vary your exercise, challenge yourself along the way, and stick to it! Be more physically active in every way. Walk into stores or restaurants instead of using the convenient drive-thru, park further away from buildings to get an extra walk in, take the stairs instead of the elevator, or play outside with your kids instead of just watching them. There are plenty of ways to get active and stay active. Your job is to implement those methods and get moving. Be sure to check with your physician before starting any type of exercise program.

GOOD TO KNOW

According to the USDA (United States Department of Agriculture) and the HHS (United States Department of Health & Human Services), poor diet and a sedentary lifestyle contribute to almost 400,000 of the 2 million annual deaths in the United States. Lack of physical activity can be linked to many health issues, including cardiovascular disease, high blood pressure, obesity, type 2 diabetes, osteoporosis, and some cancers.

Reducing Stress

The people of the Mediterranean are much more geared to a lower-stress lifestyle than we are in the United States. With our fast-paced lifestyle of parenting, working, managing our finances, and daily chores, we often become a bit more stressed than we would like to admit. This can add to a whole host of health issues, whether you realize it is happening or not. It may be time to slow down and enjoy life a bit more. Staying physically active is one thing that can help alleviate some of the stress in your life. Others might include meditation, reading a good book, listening to soothing music, doing yoga, and managing your time better. The possibilities are endless. You have to find what works for *you*.

Slow Down

Our fast-paced lifestyle often means eating meals on the run. For many, that involves a quick drive through the nearest fast-food joint, resulting in bad choices. The people of the Mediterranean tend to enjoy leisurely dining and take pleasure in all of the wonderful flavors and aromas, so a lesson in slowing down and enjoying your meals should be on your list. Slowing down when it comes to your meals can help you plan and choose your meals more wisely. You can take the time to prepare meals at home, making better choices and eating as a family. Another benefit of slowing down is that you give yourself time to think and consider not just what you are eating but how much you are eating. Did you know that slowing down can actually help satisfy your hunger at the end of the meal? You eat much less and are much more satisfied when you eat at a slower pace.

Drink Your Water

The people of the Mediterranean don't live on wine alone. Water is one of the most essential substances we can give our body. In fact, water is present in almost every cell and every part of our body. Staying properly hydrated helps your body to regulate its temperature, transport nutrients and oxygen, carry waste products, cushion joints, protect body organs, assist in the digestive process, and help to prevent constipation. The Mediterranean diet is one that is high in fiber, which means it is even more important to get the water your body needs to keep that fiber moving in the right direction. (You can read more on fiber in Chapter 15.)

Being properly hydrated can also help provide you with more energy, an improved sense of well-being, and greater endurance and stamina during physical activity. Obviously we can't live without water, and our bodies need enough to work properly. Water has no calories and is necessary to keep our bodies functioning. All that water may just be the reason for the beautiful skin on those people of the Mediterranean as well.

Because your body cannot store water, you must continually replace the water that your body loses naturally through perspiration, breathing, urination, and bowel movements. The average adult should shoot for about 8 to 12 8-ounce cups of water daily to stay properly hydrated, with people on high-fiber diets needing even a bit more. Keep in mind you do get water through foods and other beverages, but it's important to be aware of how much water you are actually drinking each day. Drink water throughout the day, keep a water bottle at your desk or in your car, drink plenty of water while exercising, and drink water at most meals.

A Common Mediterranean Diet Myth Debunked

Every diet out there has its doubters; there are always people who don't believe that a diet stands up to its claims. Even with all the research and scientific studies that prove that the principles underlying the Mediterranean style of eating are sound, you can still find a common myth: that the Mediterranean diet contains a high percentage of fat and can therefore be hazardous to your waistline and can contribute to obesity. Although the Mediterranean diet is a healthy diet, calories and portion size still matter. The fats included in this diet are heart healthy, but keep in mind that fat in general—whether healthy or not—is still high in calories.

Low-fat diets are not always the answer to permanent weight loss and good health, because it's the type of fat you eat that matters most. Just because someone follows a low-fat diet doesn't mean they are eating healthy fats. A diet can be higher in healthy fats and still be a healthy way of eating.

As long as you keep your portion sizes in check—not just with healthy fats and oils, but with all of the foods included on the diet—your waistline shouldn't have anything to worry about. If you consider all of the healthy foods you'll be eating, the decrease in unhealthy fats and foods, and the addition of more physical activity, you'll probably even lose a few pounds.

TO YOUR HEALTH

The Mediterranean diet is similar to the dietary recommendations of the American Heart Association (AHA), but they are not exactly the same. A few differences emerge with the biggest being the recommendation for fat intake. The Mediterranean diet is about 40 percent fat as opposed to the recommended 30 percent by the AHA. However, the majority of fat on the Mediterranean diet comes from healthy fat sources.

A Whole-Life Approach

This diet does not entail making drastic changes to your present eating style. In fact, what makes the Mediterranean diet so unique and so great is how practical it is in real life. It is a realistic way of life and one that you can incorporate and feel good about for a lifetime.

The health differences between people of the Mediterranean and people who consume the typical Western diet are due to their lifestyles as a whole. The Mediterranean way of life is unique in that it focuses not only on what you eat but also on your overall lifestyle—it's a whole-life approach to good health. It's a permanent solution as opposed to something one might do for a temporary period of time simply to lose weight.

Not Just a "Diet"

The Mediterranean diet is not really a "diet" at all. When we think of the word *diet* it conjures up thoughts of fad diets gone wrong, expensive weight-loss schemes, and days of deprivation.

This way of life focuses on what you *can* have instead of what you *cannot*. And what you can have are the very best, healthiest, freshest foods. That doesn't sound like the typical "diet" to me! We are not saying that one of the health benefits of a Mediterranean diet can't be shedding a few pounds, but that is not the main purpose of this so-called "diet." It's intended to be a lifestyle change.

Making It Mainstream

You don't need to live in the Mediterranean or be of Mediterranean descent to enjoy this diet and to reap its benefits. However, for the Mediterranean diet to be effective you do need to make a commitment to making this diet a permanent way of life. The Mediterranean diet is sensible and realistic, both of which are essential when it comes to something you need to follow for life.

The components of this diet work like the wheels on a car. They all need to be present to make the car go. However, not all of the tires need to match for the car to go. In other words, you don't always have to eat the traditional foods of the Mediterranean to get the most from this diet. Throughout this book, we will help you to incorporate this diet and realistically fit it into your lifestyle while still reaping all of the important health benefits.

The Least You Need to Know

- The Mediterranean diet originates from 16 different countries around this region.
- A few key components that make this diet healthy include healthy fats, fresh foods, an abundance of plant foods, physical activity, and lower stress levels.
- The Mediterranean diet incorporates many nutritional powerhouse foods that can fit realistically into anyone's life.
- The Mediterranean diet encompasses a whole-life approach.

The Good Health Diet

In This Chapter

- The connection to better heart health
- On track to a healthy weight
- Lowering your risk for cancer
- Preventing depressive disorders
- Guarding against diabetes
- Aiding in other medical conditions

If you are looking for a heart-healthy eating plan, the Mediterranean diet might just be the plan for you. However, that is far from the only health benefit this diet can provide. The Mediterranean diet boasts an impressive list of health benefits that countless people can relate to.

Did you know that you can improve your heart health, manage your weight, lower your risk for some cancers, and even improve blood sugar control by making some realistic lifestyle changes? Well, you can—and you will soon see how!

Improve Cardiovascular Health

Who says that eating a heart-healthy diet has to be tasteless? Stealing some recommendations from the Mediterranean diet and incorporating them into your everyday life can be something you can actually enjoy. The days of bland, low-fat, incredibly restrictive diets that were once recommended for heart disease prevention are gone, replaced by a colorful, fresh, and flavorful diet that amps up the healthy fats, seasonal produce, whole grains, legumes, seafood, and wonderful herbs and spices—and that is something you can most definitely sink your teeth into.

The Mediterranean diet is known as the gold standard for a heart-healthy approach. It has been researched, studied, and proven that this type of diet has a strong correlation to improved cardiovascular health. Ever since Dr. Ancel Key's famous Seven Countries Study, research supporting a Mediterranean eating pattern has been flowing in.

A study published in the *New England Journal of Medicine* in 2003 inspected at length the eating habits of more than 22,000 people living in Greece. During the intense four-year study, researchers confirmed that the closer people followed the Mediterranean diet, the less likely they were to die from either heart disease or cancer. In addition, a large clinical study sponsored by the National Institutes of Health (NIH) and the American Association of Retired Persons (AARP) published results in the Archives of Internal Medicine in 2007 suggesting that there is strong evidence that implementing a Mediterranean dietary pattern lowers the risk for death from all causes including deaths due to cardiovascular disease and cancer in the U.S. population.

Need even more proof? How about results from a study published in the *American Journal of Clinical Nutrition* in 2007 that concluded that frequent consumption of foods from the Mediterranean pattern may reduce cardiovascular disease as well as ischemic heart disease risks. Not only does the Mediterranean diet help prevent heart disease, but the Lyon Diet Heart Study, done in 2001, provided strong evidence that people eating a Mediterranean diet had a 50 to 70 percent lower risk of recurrent heart disease.

What Is Cardiovascular Disease?

The terms cardiovascular disease and heart disease are often used interchangeably. Both terms generally describe several health issues that relate to the heart and the blood vessels, including coronary heart disease (heart attack and/or stroke), angina (chest pain), and heart failure.

Cardiovascular disease (CVD) is the number one killer of both men and women in the United States. According to the American Heart Association, an estimated 80 million American adults (one in three) have one or more forms of cardiovascular disease. Looking at the most recent statistics, CVD claimed over 800,000 lives in 2006—about 34 percent of all deaths. In 2009, it was estimated that heart disease cost the United States over $300 billion. Do these statistics startle you? They should, but the good news is there *is* something you can do to avoid becoming one of the statistics. Making smarter dietary and lifestyle choices can put you on the road to better heart health.

Are You at Risk?

Two risk factors that we don't have any control over are age and genetics. Your risk increases as you get older, and a strong family history can put you at risk. Other risk factors include *low-density lipoprotein (LDL)* or "bad" cholesterol, high *triglycerides*, high blood pressure, and *high-density lipoprotein (HDL)* or "good" cholesterol. In addition you could be putting yourself at risk if you are sedentary, are overweight or obese, have uncontrolled diabetes, drink alcohol excessively, consume a poor diet, and/or have high stress levels. Do any of these apply to you? If so, it may be time to take a serious look at your diet and lifestyle.

DEFINITION

Triglycerides are the main form of fat in foods. Excess calories from any type of food source are processed in the body and changed to triglycerides for storage as fat in the body. Normal triglyceride levels should be less than 150 mg/dL. **Low-density lipoprotein (LDL),** or "bad" cholesterol, causes cholesterol buildup in artery walls, which can put you at risk for heart disease and stroke. On the contrary, **high-density lipoprotein (HDL),** or "good" cholesterol, protects you from heart disease by ridding your body of dietary cholesterol.

How Does the Mediterranean Diet Help?

The good news is that, even with most risk factors, many forms of heart disease can be prevented and treated with both diet and exercise. That is where the Mediterranean diet comes in. Key components of this diet make it able to help prevent and even reverse some major health problems.

The Cholesterol Connection

Blood cholesterol levels are a significant risk factor for heart disease. The higher your cholesterol level, both total and LDL, the higher your risk for heart disease. Therefore it is vital to have your cholesterol tested on a regular basis. You should know what your personal numbers are so that you understand this all-important risk factor. Knowing your levels for total cholesterol, as well as LDL and HDL, tells you whether your blood cholesterol is putting you at risk for heart disease and/or stroke.

As we have mentioned, cholesterol comes in two basic forms: LDL (or bad) cholesterol and HDL (or good) cholesterol. When LDL, or low-density lipoprotein, and total cholesterol are too high, it causes cholesterol (or plaque) to build up in the walls of your arteries. This condition is known as atherosclerosis, or hardening of the arteries, and it puts you at higher risk for heart disease. HDL, or high-density lipoprotein, rids your body of cholesterol by taking it from the artery walls and sending it to the liver for removal from the body, giving your heart some protection. Your total cholesterol level should be less than 200 mg/dL to be at a desirable level. LDL cholesterol should be less than 100 mg/dL, with HDL being above 60 mg/dL to offer any heart protection. Cholesterol testing should be done after fasting for at least 12 hours. Your doctor can determine how often you should get your cholesterol tested.

With the Mediterranean diet's combination of high fiber (especially soluble fiber), low amounts of saturated and trans fats, high consumption of unsaturated fats (especially monounsaturated fats), and physical activity, it has been concluded that this diet can modestly lower LDL and raise HDL cholesterol. In addition it has been shown to decrease triglyceride levels, another possible risk factor for heart disease.

HEALTHY MORSELS

Plant stanols and sterols are found naturally in fruits, vegetables, and plant oils and have been found to lower LDL cholesterol. They work by inhibiting the absorption of cholesterol in the body. Because the Mediterranean diet is abundant in fruits and vegetables, it provides a natural LDL-lowering effect.

Aid in Weight Management

We have all heard the great debate about which is the best way to lose weight. No wonder folks are so confused! Is it low fat, high fat, no carbs, high protein, low protein, no sugar, good fat? As it turns out, there is no one "best way" to lose weight. However, the eating style of the Mediterranean is catching on as a realistic and healthy way to shed some pounds.

Most of us know that to lose weight and keep it off you need to permanently change your lifestyle. The Mediterranean diet encompasses this whole-life approach. With its healthy food choices, moderate consumption of foods, and physical activity—a change to this type of lifestyle can help you to maintain a healthier weight.

A recent study published in the *New England Journal of Medicine* revealed that a calorie-controlled Mediterranean diet could be more effective for weight loss than a low-fat diet, while also offering additional health benefits. The Mediterranean diet is not a quick fix to your weight problems; however, by conforming to this type of lifestyle, you may see your waistline begin to slowly shrink. With the good habits you establish, and the bad ones you throw away, it is bound to happen—not to mention that it can be empowering to make positive changes in your life and have control over the way you are living it. That is a great motivator!

The Dangers of Obesity

The prevalence of obesity in the United States is truly staggering. The most recent study done by the U.S. Centers for Disease Control and Prevention (CDC) showed that a whopping 32 percent of American adults are overweight and 34 percent are obese. Being overweight or obese has many dangers. Research has shown that being overweight or obese increases one's risk for the following conditions:

- Coronary heart disease
- Type 2 diabetes
- Breast, colon, and endometrial cancers
- High blood pressure (hypertension)
- High cholesterol and/or triglyceride levels
- Stroke
- Liver and gallbladder disease
- Sleep apnea and other respiratory problems
- Osteoarthritis
- Gynecological problems

There are countless reasons to choose a lifestyle that will not only increase your health but also help you to shed excess weight. Given the statistics, it is obvious that the traditional Western diet leaves much to be desired! This is where the Mediterranean diet comes in. Not only can this diet help you manage your weight, but many of the health problems that are caused by obesity are the exact problems that can be treated, prevented, or reversed by following the Mediterranean diet.

What Should You Weigh?

Not quite sure if you are obese, overweight, or at a normal weight? Not quite sure if your weight puts you at health risks? Not quite sure what you should weigh? Now is the time to find out.

For adults, Body Mass Index, or BMI, is used to screen for weight categories that may lead to health risks. BMI is determined by using weight and height to calculate a number or index. You can easily calculate your BMI by visiting www.nhlbisupport. com/bmi/, or you can use the following formula:

Weight (pounds) ÷ height (inches) squared × 703

For example, if you weigh 160 pounds and have a height of 5'7" (67"), you would calculate your BMI this way:

160 ÷ (67) squared × 703 = 25.05

Once you know your BMI, you can determine your weight category:

- Underweight = BMI of less than 18.5
- Normal weight = BMI of 18.5 – 24.9
- Overweight = BMI of 25 – 29.9
- Obese = BMI of 30 or greater

TO YOUR HEALTH

Figuring your BMI is not a direct measure of body fat. As a result, some folks such as athletes or body builders who carry extra weight due to more muscle may be classified as overweight or obese even though they do not have excess body fat.

Cancer Protection

Cancer is the second leading cause of death in the United States behind heart disease, so it's no surprise that most of us will perk up and listen when we hear that something may help to lower our cancer risk.

Studies show that the overall cancer incidence in people following a Mediterranean-type eating pattern is much lower than those not following it. In 2008, the *British Journal of Cancer* concluded from a general population investigation that adherence to the traditional Mediterranean diet is associated with markedly and significantly reduced incidence of overall cancer, and this reduced incidence was appreciably larger than predicted from examining individual Mediterranean diet components. This is evidence that it's the diet as a whole, and the many cancer-fighting foods included in the diet, working to provide protection.

It has been estimated that close to 25 percent of colorectal cancer; 15 percent of breast cancer; and 10 percent of prostate, pancreatic, and endometrial cancers could possibly be prevented by shifting to an eating style like the Mediterranean diet. This would include changes such as eating more fruits and vegetables as well as nuts and legumes, reducing consumption of red meat and refined starches, and using more olive oil and other unsaturated fats as opposed to saturated ones. All of these are realistic lifestyle changes that can arm you with one more weapon in the battle against cancer.

Preventing Depression

Depressive disorders are serious and affect almost 18.8 million American adults—about 9.5 percent of the U.S. population. Recent research is beginning to suggest that people who follow a traditional Mediterranean diet may be less likely to develop depression. Researchers believe that these findings are based on the foods and the components of those foods, including vitamins, minerals, antioxidants, and phytonutrients.

A new study published in the *Archives of General Psychiatry* concluded that those people who most closely followed the Mediterranean diet were more than 30 percent less likely to develop depression than those people who adhered to the diet the least.

Although researchers aren't exactly clear just yet on how the foods of the Mediterranean actually help fight depression, they do believe that individual components of the diet may help to improve blood vessel function, fight inflammation, reduce the risk for heart disease, and repair oxygen-related cell damage—all of which may affect a person's risk for developing depression. It could be many components of the diet working together synergistically to add a degree of protection. These components may include omega-3 fatty acids; other unsaturated fatty acids; antioxidants from olive oil and nuts; large amounts of natural folates and other B vitamins; and flavonoids and other *phytochemicals* from fruits, vegetables, and other plant foods. The research continues on the diet's connection to depression, so stay tuned!

DEFINITION

Phytochemicals, also known as phytonutrients, are naturally occurring compounds found in plant-based foods that offer potential health benefits.

Take Control of Diabetes

New research has shown that the Mediterranean diet may be a winning solution for people with type 2 diabetes. This type of eating style may help to manage type 2 diabetes without medication, or with lower levels of medication, than following a typical low-fat diet. A recent study showed that after four years, 44 percent of people with type 2 diabetes who had never been treated with medications and were assigned to follow a calorie-controlled Mediterranean diet eventually needed diabetes medications such as pills or insulin. However, 70 percent of those who followed a low-fat diet, based on the American Heart Association guidelines, needed medications to eventually control their blood sugar. Although both diets were beneficial, the Mediterranean diet group had better blood sugar control and was much less likely to need the intervention of medications to get their blood sugars within a normal range.

These results reinforce the message that the benefits of lifestyle interventions, including diet, are essential and should not be overlooked for diabetes intervention. Although a Mediterranean diet is not the magic cure, it has plenty of features that can help to control diabetes and help people to avoid or reduce medication use.

GOOD TO KNOW

Always check with your doctor before stopping or reducing any type of medication for diabetes. Diet and lifestyle changes can help, but your doctor should decide whether diet alone is enough to control your diabetes. Keeping blood sugar in check can mean the difference between a healthy life and one with serious health issues.

Types of Diabetes

The term diabetes refers to a group of diseases that are marked by high levels of blood glucose or blood sugar due to defects in the production or action of insulin, a hormone produced in the pancreas. There are three basic forms of diabetes: type 1, type 2, and gestational (during pregnancy). Type 2 diabetes is the most common form with an estimated 20 million Americans being affected and many more that are at high risk.

With type 2 diabetes, the body does not produce enough insulin, which is needed by the body to use glucose for energy. When we eat food, our body breaks down sugars and starches into glucose, which is the main fuel for our body's cells. It is the job of insulin to take the sugar from the blood into the cells. When there is not enough insulin to do the job, glucose builds up in the blood instead of entering the cells, causing high blood sugar levels. This can lead to complications if not treated properly. Treatment can include diet and exercise modifications, oral medications, or insulin injections. Treatment is modified for each individual and their own personal needs in order to manage their blood sugars.

Diabetes can lead to a host of serious health complications, especially if it is not controlled. These include heart disease, stroke, high blood pressure, blindness, kidney disease, diseases of the nervous system, amputation, and even death.

HEALTHY MORSELS

Unlike type 2 diabetes where the body doesn't produce enough insulin, type 1 diabetes is caused when the body produces *no* insulin, and these people need insulin injections to survive. Type 1 diabetes is much less common than type 2 diabetes and cannot be treated with diet and lifestyle changes alone.

Are You at Risk?

People with uncontrolled diabetes can be at risk for serious health conditions. Therefore it is important to know if you have diabetes, or are at risk for it, so that you can take the proper precautions. People who are overweight or obese, have a family history of diabetes, and/or are physically inactive have a higher risk for type 2 diabetes. Other risk factors include high blood pressure, high LDL cholesterol, low HDL cholesterol, high triglyceride levels, cardiovascular disease, history of gestational diabetes, and abnormal fasting glucose levels (blood sugar levels taken when not eating for a prolonged period of time). Ethnicity can also play a role in determining your risk.

People with diabetes are at a higher risk for heart attacks, strokes, and high blood pressure, so it's vital that their lifestyle not only be aimed at stringent blood sugar control but also at other health aspects. Following the Mediterranean diet has been proven to help control blood sugar, but for diabetics it can be particularly important since it is also a heart-healthy way of life.

Connection to Other Health Issues

To really soak up all that the Mediterranean diet has to offer, it's essential to look at all of its benefits. As more research is done, more health benefits are being revealed about the Mediterranean way of life.

> **GOOD TO KNOW**
>
> Although the Mediterranean diet may help ward off some serious health conditions, it is important not to diagnose or treat yourself for any type of medical condition you might have—or think you have. Leave it up to the experts and always check with your doctor for proper diagnosis and treatment. However, don't be afraid to bring up the benefits of a Mediterranean lifestyle with your doctor!

Hypertension

In today's hectic and chaotic society, it is not surprising that hypertension is becoming all too common. With the number of Americans who are overweight or obese, eat unhealthy diets, are physically inactive, and experience high stress levels, problems with high blood pressure will likely continue to be a reality.

Blood pressure is the force of blood against the walls of your arteries. When your blood pressure is elevated over time, it is diagnosed as hypertension or high blood pressure. Hypertension makes your heart work too hard and can increase your risk for a host of serious health issues including heart and artery damage, stroke, kidney disease, and vision loss. These are not symptoms of high blood pressure, because this disease really has no symptoms or warning signs. Your risk for health issues increase even more if, along with high blood pressure, you smoke, are overweight or obese, have high cholesterol, have diabetes, are physically inactive, are male, are older, or have a genetic predisposition. Anyone can develop high blood pressure, and it's estimated that one in every four Americans has high blood pressure.

Even though hypertension does have strong genetic links, plenty of evidence confirms that good nutrition and a healthy lifestyle can delay or prevent the onset of hypertension as well as treat it. When it comes to both preventing and treating hypertension, many people today look to natural alternatives.

Could the Mediterranean diet be the answer for many? According to a 2008 study published in the *European Journal of Clinical Nutrition*, the Mediterranean style of eating may hold some promise in helping to prevent hypertension. This is not the only study that has been published that recognizes this diet's potential for high blood pressure prevention. Another was published in 2004 in the *American Journal of Clinical Nutrition* demonstrating that blood pressure levels were lower in those people who followed a Mediterranean diet. This particular study highlighted the importance of olive oil in proportion to blood pressure decreases. The bottom line is that even though a Mediterranean eating style may not be 100 percent effective for all people, especially those at high risk of hypertension due to family history, it could delay its onset and possibly reduce the amount of medication that is needed for treatment.

GOOD TO KNOW

A blood pressure level of 140/90 mmHg or higher is considered high. If your blood pressure is between 120/80 mmHg and 139/89 mmHg, you have pre-hypertension, meaning you are likely to develop high blood pressure. Have your blood pressure checked regularly.

Alzheimer's Disease

Alzheimer's disease is a brain disorder and the most common form of dementia, which is a general term used for memory loss and loss of other intellectual abilities. It is estimated that 5.3 million Americans are living with this disease. It is a progressive disease and is eventually fatal. There is currently no cure.

Studies suggest that following a Mediterranean diet can lower the risk for mental decline, and adding exercise can lower your risk even more. A 2006 study by the Taub Institute for Research on Alzheimer's Disease and the Aging Brain at Columbia University Medical Center showed that elderly people from one specific state whose eating habits most resembled the Mediterranean diet had nearly a 40 percent lower risk of Alzheimer's disease compared to those with poor diets. In addition, the study showed that those who were more physically active had the least risk for Alzheimer's disease.

It doesn't seem to be a matter of eating less and exercising more, but rather one of eating well and staying physically active. It's important to remember that the Mediterranean diet and exercise may not completely protect a person against Alzheimer's disease and cognitive decline, but it may help to lower one's risk.

Parkinson's Disease

Parkinson's disease is a degenerative disorder that affects the central nervous system, often impairing motor skills, speech, and other functions. It is a chronic and progressive disease, meaning that it persists for a lifetime and symptoms become worse with time. There is presently no cure for Parkinson's disease, but there are medications that can help dramatically relieve symptoms for most sufferers.

Through the many studies done on the Mediterranean diet, it has become evident that the incidence of Parkinson's disease is lower in people that adhere to a Mediterranean eating style. In 2007, a study published in the *American Journal of Clinical Nutrition* concluded that dietary patterns with high intake of fruits, vegetables, legumes, whole grains, nuts, fish, and poultry combined with a low intake of saturated fat and a moderate intake of alcohol may help protect against Parkinson's disease. Does that diet sound familiar? Well, it should—that's the Mediterranean diet in a nutshell.

Rheumatoid Arthritis

People who are diagnosed with rheumatoid arthritis suffer from painful swelling, mostly in the joints of the hands and feet. Rheumatoid arthritis is an autoimmune disorder, meaning that it occurs because your immune system mistakenly attacks your own body's tissues. There is currently no cure for this type of arthritis, but there have been advances in treatment options in the past few decades.

It seems that there is some connection between rheumatoid arthritis and the Mediterranean diet. The diet has been shown to positively benefit people with arthritis by reducing inflammation and improving function. The results of a 2003 study in the *Annals of Rheumatic Diseases* indicated that by adjusting to a Mediterranean diet, patients with rheumatoid arthritis obtained a reduction in inflammatory activity, an increase in physical function, and improved vitality. This is not to say that the diet will cure or dramatically improve a person's symptoms, but it does seem that there is a modest benefit for arthritis sufferers.

The Least You Need to Know

- The Mediterranean diet has been a proven ally in helping to lower the risk for heart disease.
- Weight loss is possible with a calorie-controlled Mediterranean eating plan.
- The risk of some types of cancer could be lowered by following the Mediterranean way of life.
- The Mediterranean diet is a tool to help type 2 diabetics control blood sugar and possibly reduce medication use.
- Studies show that the Mediterranean diet may be beneficial for other medical conditions such as depression, hypertension, Alzheimer's disease, Parkinson's disease, and rheumatoid arthritis.

Components of the Mediterranean Diet

In This Chapter

- All about the Mediterranean Diet Pyramid
- A closer look at the food groups on the Mediterranean Diet Pyramid
- The EatWise Pyramid and the USDA's MyPyramid
- How the food pyramids compare
- Which pyramid should you choose?

The Mediterranean diet is about an eating pattern. It's much more than any one single food that generates health benefits and longevity. Instead it revolves around how particular healthy cuisine involving all of the food groups and a healthier life-style work cohesively to construct the diet and make it what it is. The Mediterranean Diet Pyramid puts this all together in one neat, visual package.

The Mediterranean Diet Pyramid

Since the Mediterranean Diet Pyramid was first introduced in 1993, many people have taken notice. Many restaurants, chefs, cookbooks, weight-loss companies, and health professionals have willingly embraced this way of meal planning and eating. The Mediterranean Diet Pyramid was developed as a way to help people visualize the diet by using a graphic to represent it.

The Oldways Preservation & Exchange Trust, along with the Harvard School of Public Health and the World Health Organization, introduced the diet and the pyramid 17 years ago at a conference in Cambridge, Massachusetts. The pyramid has remained a universally recognized guide to the Mediterranean style of eating. The pyramid was created using the most current science-based research to symbolize the traditional Mediterranean diet. The pyramid not only represents the foods of the Mediterranean but takes into account other factors that come highly recommended as part of the lifestyle including physical activity, the enjoyment of meals with others, and the appreciation for the pleasure of eating these tasty and healthy foods.

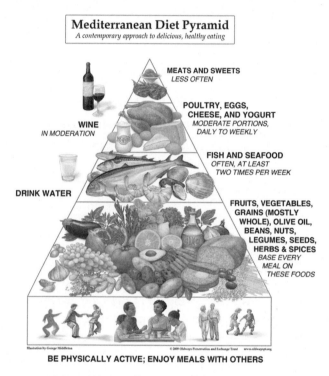

Used by permission, © 2009 Oldways Preservation & Exchange Trust, www.oldwayspt.org.

A Few Changes

Since its initial development in 1993, the pyramid has undergone some renovations to reflect the latest research findings and ongoing studies. During the 15th anniversary of the Mediterranean Diet Conference (where the diet and pyramid were first introduced), updates were made by the Scientific Advisory Board to provide some beneficial improvements.

The major changes made to the pyramid include:

- The grouping together of all plant foods including fruits, vegetables, grains, nuts, legumes, seeds, olives, and olive oil. This group now encompasses the largest section of the pyramid. This change was made to draw direct attention to the key role plant foods play in good health.

- The addition of herbs and spices to the pyramid. These enhance flavor and aroma and reduce the need for fat and salt in cooking.

- The emphasis of eating more fish and shellfish. Consume these foods at least twice per week in order to obtain their unique health benefits.

Explaining the Pyramid

The Mediterranean Diet Pyramid is an easy-to-follow visual aid to help people implement the Mediterranean diet. The pyramid is arranged in a way that suggests how often certain types of foods should be consumed in order to get the most health benefits. The base of the pyramid shows foods to consume more often; as you move up the pyramid, it shows foods to eat less often. While changes were recently made to the pyramid, it still emphasizes:

- Be physically active as much as possible and enjoy meals with others as the foundation of this type of healthy lifestyle.
- Choose the least-processed forms of plant foods.
- Use olive oil for most cooking, baking, salad dressings, and vegetables.
- Consume low-fat or fat-free cheeses and yogurts in moderation.
- Consume poultry more often than red meats.
- Drink red wine in moderation (or purple grape juice, if you don't drink wine).
- Drink water. It's essential for life and proper hydration, which contributes to good health, a sense of well-being, and higher energy levels.
- Eat in moderation.

TO YOUR HEALTH

The Mediterranean Diet Pyramid doesn't get specific with serving sizes and instead only shows how often certain foods should be consumed. Portion size is still important, so always employ the notion of moderation.

The Plant Group

Recent changes to the Mediterranean Diet Pyramid make the plant group the largest group. This group of foods is at the bottom of the pyramid, above physical activity and enjoying meals with others, signifying that it is one of the essential foundations of this eating style. It now incorporates *all* plant foods including fruits, vegetables, grains (mostly whole), olives and olive oil, beans, nuts and seeds, legumes, and herbs and spices.

Guidelines for the plant group specify basing every meal on these foods. This group is an important source of fiber, vitamins, minerals, antioxidants, phytonutrients, and energy. An eating pattern that is based on these foods promotes good health and even weight control when chosen wisely and eaten in moderation. Because the foods in this group are at the bottom of the pyramid, they tend to be eaten in larger amounts and more frequently, so keep and continue to be aware of portion sizes. The guidelines also call for eating seasonally fresh foods and locally grown foods when possible.

Fruits and Vegetables

There is a vast variety of produce that is popular in the Mediterranean region, and because they are frequently eaten in season, they may be fresher and more nutritious. Shop the perimeter of the grocery store where most of the fresh foods are located, and try out local farmers' markets in your area. Although the pyramid doesn't specify serving sizes, it is recommended that your goal be to aim for at least 7 to 9 servings of a variety of high-fiber fruits and vegetables daily. Don't worry, you don't need to eat fruits and vegetables straight from the Mediterranean or even rely on only the most popular ones. Finding produce that is in season in your area and that you enjoy is the most important point to remember.

TO YOUR HEALTH

Dried fruits such as prunes, dates, cranberries, figs, raisins, and apricots are very high in fiber and can be easy to find and store all year long. Try them in salads, rice dishes, homemade breads, casseroles, and desserts.

Grains

No carb phobias here! Grains are chock full of carbohydrates and are our body's main source of energy, fiber, vitamins, and minerals. The Mediterranean diet includes plenty of whole grains that are as minimally processed as possible. The less processed they are, the more nutrition they retain. Whole grains include whole-wheat bread, whole-grain cereal, brown rice, couscous, bulgur, oatmeal, polenta, and quinoa.

Olives and Olive Oil

When most people think of the Mediterranean diet, it's usually olives and olive oil that first come to mind. Almost everything is cooked with healthier oils such as olive oil (the most popular), and olives are served quite often at meals throughout the day. Olive oil is the chief source of dietary fat used for most cooking, baking, and salad dressings. Extra-virgin olive oil is highest in the healthy monounsaturated fats, phytonutrients, and other essential nutrients. To transform your diet, begin to replace the oil you now use with olive oil. Replace your butter, margarine, and/or salad dressings with olive oil. Rather than use margarine or butter on your bread, try dipping it in olive oil!

Beans, Nuts, Legumes, and Seeds

Beans, nuts, legumes, and seeds are all good sources of healthy fats, fiber, and even protein. They add unique flavor and texture to popular Mediterranean dishes. You can add beans and legumes to all types of dishes, and in the Mediterranean they are often the center of the daily main meal. In addition, nuts and seeds make great snacks and are often used in desserts. Because nuts are high in fat—although healthy fat—they can be high in calories, so eat in moderation (as in a handful of nuts daily).

Herbs and Spices

Herbs (fresh or dried) and spices have always been used abundantly throughout the Mediterranean; however, they are a recent addition to the Mediterranean Diet Pyramid. Herbs and spices such as oregano, rosemary, red pepper, garlic, and mint add flavor and aroma to foods and can reduce or even eliminate the need to add salt or fat when cooking. They can help to bring out the natural flavor of foods, and many are rich in health-promoting antioxidants. Herbs and spices directly contribute to the exclusive identity of various Mediterranean cuisine and dishes.

Fish and Seafood

The next step up on the Mediterranean Diet Pyramid is the fish and seafood group. It's not surprising that fish and shellfish are so popular; the Mediterranean regions are surrounded by coastlines. Fish and shellfish are sources of healthy lean protein and heart-healthy fats in the form of omega-3 fatty acids. Fish is not just heart healthy—recent research shows that eating fish can help to reduce the cognitive decline that can come with aging, so eat up! Time to drop the "But I don't like fish!" excuse and give it a try. There are many varieties to choose from, and they all have their own distinct flavors.

The guidelines for seafood are a new part of the Mediterranean Diet Pyramid. The guiding principle on this food group is to consume them at least twice a week.

> **TO YOUR HEALTH**
>
> In the Mediterranean, fish and shellfish are commonly cooked in stews or steamed rather than battered and fried. Fish cooks quickly and can make for quick and easy meals.

All types of fish and shellfish are included in this category, but it's the fattier fish that are most popular, including tuna, herring, sardines, and salmon. The fattier the fish, the healthier they are because their fat source is heart healthy. (See Chapter 14 for more information on these fat sources and their health benefits.) Shellfish such as mussels, clams, and shrimp also have similar benefits and are popular.

Cheese and Yogurt

As we continue to travel up the Mediterranean Diet Pyramid, the cheese and yogurt group is the next stop. The calcium and vitamin D found in cheese and yogurt is essential for strong bones and a healthy heart. These dairy foods are also wonderful sources of protein. Cheese and yogurt are eaten often in the traditional Mediterranean diet, but you don't need to limit this group to those two foods. Low-fat or fat-free milk and other dairy products are also great sources of protein, calcium, and vitamin D and can definitely fit into this group.

The guidelines of the pyramid specifically state that moderate portions should be consumed on a daily or weekly basis. Low-fat and nonfat dairy products are recommended. Avoid sugary yogurts and stick to plain or Greek yogurts. For a touch of sweetness, try adding a bit of honey.

Poultry and Eggs

One more step up the pyramid is poultry and eggs, which are another important source of high-quality protein. However, as we move up the pyramid, the sections become smaller, signifying the need for lower consumption. The guidelines of the pyramid state that poultry and eggs should be eaten in moderate portions every two days or weekly. Eggs are used commonly in cooking and baking and it is recommended to consume no more than seven eggs per week. When consuming poultry, stick with the white meat and remove the skin to lower saturated fat and cholesterol content.

Meats and Sweets

Meats and sweets top the pyramid, meaning that you should consume these least. Sweets are not all that popular in the Mediterranean and are usually consumed only in small portions. Fresh fruit and/or nuts are commonly eaten to end a meal instead of a sugar-laden dessert. Gelato and sorbet in small portions are popular and sometimes consumed a few times per week.

When the pyramid refers to meats in this section, it's essentially singling out red meats. There isn't much room for red meats in this diet, which are high in saturated fat and cholesterol—and therefore bad for your heart. Red meat is consumed only a few times per month, with a recommendation to eat no more than 12 to 16 ounces monthly. Leaner cuts are preferred, and you should always trim away any visible fat. Still have a taste for a burger? Try ground turkey breast and add a slice of avocado, slice of tomato, and a dab of olive oil. You won't even miss the red meat!

Wine

Wine is a part of the pyramid because it is a normal part of the Mediterranean lifestyle. It is consumed quite regularly, but moderately, with meals in the Mediterranean. Red wine has more nutritional benefits than you might realize. Women can include one five-ounce serving per day and men can include two five-ounce servings daily. Of course, individuals should only drink wine if they are medically able to do so and are of age. Purple grape juice makes a great alternative.

GOOD TO KNOW

The updated Mediterranean Diet Pyramid and associated recommendations are reliable for most adults. However, children, pregnant women, and those with special dietary needs may require supplementation as well as modifications. Always check with your doctor before starting a new diet plan.

The EatWise Pyramid

The EatWise Pyramid was also developed by the Oldways Preservation & Exchange Trust and experts from Harvard School of Public Health. This pyramid is modeled after the original Mediterranean Diet Pyramid. It is a visualization of the EatWise Guidelines, developed by Oldways along with world leaders in food science, behavior change, and culinary expertise.

The EatWise Guidelines were developed to help teach people how to "eat wise" based on the basic principles of the Mediterranean diet, but they are more geared toward the USDA Dietary Guidelines for Americans by using more familiar foods. The EatWise Guidelines were developed because people were not following the existing USDA Dietary Guidelines and that those guidelines were not persuading people to change their bad habits. Oldways believes that the EatWise Guidelines are practical, down-to-earth, and realistic and that they will help individuals and families focus on lifestyle habits that result in lifelong good health.

The EatWise Pyramid is set up slightly differently than the Mediterranean Diet Pyramid. However, both pyramids emphasize eating a balanced diet, drinking plenty of water, getting regular physical activity, and drinking alcohol in moderation. The EatWise Pyramid is another effective way to help you visualize the Mediterranean diet and make it part of your everyday life. Find out more about it at www.oldwayspt.org.

The USDA's MyPyramid

In 2005, the USDA changed its Food Guide Pyramid concept to the MyPyramid Food Guidance System. The MyPyramid graphic is meant to help people visualize the *Dietary Guidelines for Americans.* It is similar to the way that the Mediterranean Diet Pyramid helps people to visualize the concepts of the Mediterranean diet. MyPyramid has a new look with six colored bands that represent the food groups: grains (orange), vegetables (green), fruits (red), milk (blue), meats/beans (purple), and fats/oils (yellow). MyPyramid does not display individual foods or numbers of servings per food group on the actual graphic. Instead, the graphic is meant to lead individuals to the website for a more interactive experience; go to www.mypyramid.gov.

DEFINITION

The **Dietary Guidelines for Americans** are science- and evidence-based nutritional and fitness goals that promote health and reduce the risk of chronic disease. The advice is meant to guide people to eat a healthier diet.

The MyPyramid graphic holds several key messages:

- The figure climbing the pyramid represents the importance of daily physical activity.

- The words "Steps to a Healthier You" suggest that health benefits can be made by taking small steps to improve your diet and lifestyle.

- Each of the six colored bands indicate a different food group and suggests that you should eat a variety of foods each day.

- Each band on the pyramid has a different width showing the relative amounts of food a person should choose from each food group.

Comparing the Pyramids

The most basic difference between MyPyramid and the Mediterranean Diet Pyramid is that one focuses on common foods of the United States and the other focuses on the cuisine of the Mediterranean regions. However, there are several similarities that can be found between the two pyramids and styles of eating. Both eating patterns recommend consuming a variety of fruits, vegetables, and whole grains; choosing low-fat or fat-free dairy products; choosing lean proteins; eating sweets less often; and including physical activity.

HEALTHY MORSELS

Oldways, the developer of the Mediterranean Diet Pyramid, had input into the development of MyPyramid and the most recent Dietary Guidelines for Americans. It looks like Oldways and the USDA are slowly but surely beginning to work together for the health of all.

Some general differences include:

- MyPyramid groups meats and other proteins together and recommends eating leaner cuts of meat. The Mediterranean Diet Pyramid separates red meats, seafood, and poultry and eggs. Red meat is recommended much less and fish is emphasized more.

- MyPyramid recommends limiting fat intake. The Mediterranean Diet Pyramid emphasizes more use of healthy fats—specifically olive oil, which is grouped with plant foods.

- The Mediterranean Diet Pyramid was designed to illustrate proportions rather than specific amounts or serving sizes of foods, recommending only how often to eat certain foods. Detailed information on serving sizes and number of servings are not provided as they are in the MyPyramid online system or the Dietary Guidelines for Americans.

- Wine is an illustrated and recommended part of the Mediterranean Diet Pyramid.

Making Your Choice

Even though there are some differences between the USDA's MyPyramid and the Mediterranean Diet Pyramid, the one common goal they both have is to guide people to a healthier eating style and a more beneficial way of life. MyPyramid is based on American eating patterns with flexibility in food choices being an important objective. Thus a person can easily choose to eat in a Mediterranean style by choosing foods common to that region, within the framework of the USDA's MyPyramid. If you are a die-hard Mediterranean fan, utilizing the Mediterranean Diet Pyramid can be highly beneficial in helping you to reach your health goals. So the choice is yours—whichever helps you to reach your goals and stick with them is the right choice to make.

Keep in mind that a healthy and balanced diet will accommodate most foods and drinks; as long as you practice moderation and make wise choices most of the time, you will be okay. Enjoy a steak or a piece of birthday cake occasionally—these are all parts of a realistic lifestyle and can be part of a healthy lifestyle.

The Least You Need to Know

- Oldways, the Harvard School of Public Health, and the World Health Organization first introduced the Mediterranean Diet Pyramid, along with the actual Mediterranean diet concept, in 1993.
- The Mediterranean Diet Pyramid is a visualization of the Mediterranean diet.
- In 2008, the Mediterranean Diet Pyramid was revised to reflect a few beneficial changes.
- The Mediterranean Diet Pyramid shows you which foods to eat more often and which foods to eat less often. In addition, it recommends including physical activity and enjoying meals with others as an important part of the Mediterranean lifestyle.
- Both the Mediterranean Diet Pyramid and the USDA's MyPyramid promote healthy diets though they have some notable differences.

The Basics of the Mediterranean Diet

How does the Mediterranean diet compare with all of the different types of diets out there? This part gives you a pretty good idea of how this diet stacks up against some of the more popular diets out there, including the Atkins diet and the South Beach diet. And when you have no doubt that the Mediterranean diet is for you, we teach you how to fit this way of eating into your lifestyle. This part gets to the heart of the matter and takes a closer look at the essential foods and food groups from the Mediterranean Diet Pyramid. We will cover all of the foods and beverages you need to embrace, from olive oil to fruits and veggies to whole grains—focusing on how, what, and why.

How Other Diets Stack Up

In This Chapter

- Is the Mediterranean diet as healthy as the American Heart Association recommendations?
- Other heart-healthy weight-loss diets reviewed
- Carbs aren't always the enemy
- Losing weight with the right motivation and commitment

Everyone is interested in being healthy and living longer. And as luck may have it, there are scores of different diets out there for those seeking help, whether it is to become healthier or shed some unwanted pounds. The problem is that there are almost too many choices, and it can become a daunting task. People often don't know where to turn. Countless diets pat themselves on the back for being the best and the most effective. They all have their own health and weight-loss claims, but some are safer and more effective than others.

What do the experts say about the Mediterranean diet? According to years of studies and research, the Mediterranean diet is, without doubt, a healthy way of life. Renowned medical journals, professional health organizations, and doctors from all walks of life have agreed that the Mediterranean diet has what it takes to improve health for many. Whatever your reason for adopting a new way of eating, you should always do your homework before making such an important decision.

The American Heart Association's Heart-Healthy Diet

When you think of a heart-healthy diet, you might assume that the American Heart Association (AHA) is the leader of the pack. The AHA is a national voluntary health agency whose mission is to help people lower their risk of cardiovascular diseases and stroke and to live healthier lives. Like the Mediterranean diet, the recommendations and guidelines of the AHA's heart-healthy diet are proven through years of studies and research.

Guidelines

The Mediterranean style of eating closely resembles that of the dietary recommendations of the AHA. The biggest difference is the higher percentage of healthy fat on the Mediterranean diet. The AHA diet recommends limiting total fat to about 25 to 35 percent of your total calories and is considered to be more of a low-fat diet. The Mediterranean diet is a bit higher in fat, with about 35 to 40 percent of total calories from fat. However, even though total fat differs slightly, both diets are low in unhealthy fats, such as saturated fats and trans fats, and high in healthy fats, such as monounsaturated and polyunsaturated fats.

If you take a close look at the guidelines, you can determine just how similar these two diets really are:

- The AHA recommends limiting the amount of saturated fat (less then 7 percent of total daily calorie intake), trans fat (less then 1 percent of total daily calorie intake), and cholesterol (less than 300 mg daily) that you consume. The Mediterranean diet is naturally low in all three because it recommends limiting whole-fat dairy products, red meats, eggs, processed foods, baked goods, and fried foods. This diet also eliminates butter and/or margarines, both of which can be high in saturated fats, trans fats, and/or cholesterol.

- The AHA recommends cutting back on foods and beverages with high sugar content and/or added sugars. The Mediterranean diet is low in added sugars. People who follow this diet eat very few sweets and eat more foods that are naturally sweet, such as fruit.

- The AHA recommends choosing and preparing foods with little to no salt. This helps to lower the risk for high blood pressure and may help to control it. The Mediterranean diet is naturally low in sodium because it includes very few processed foods. Most foods are consumed in their natural forms or made from scratch. In addition, in place of salt, herbs and spices are used abundantly in cooking.

HEALTHY MORSELS

The AHA goal for all people is to eat less than 1,500 mg of sodium per day (based on a 2,000 calorie diet). Currently, Americans consume on average 3,400 mg daily, twice what is recommended.

- The AHA recommends keeping a check on your calorie intake and for healthy adults, aiming for at least 30 minutes of moderate intensity physical activity at least five days per week to help maintain a healthy weight and develop cardiovascular fitness. One of the main foundations of the Mediterranean diet is physical activity.

- The AHA recommends eating at least 25 grams of dietary fiber every day, preferably from food sources such as whole grains, fruits, vegetables, and legumes as opposed to supplements. All of these foods are included in the largest part of the Mediterranean Diet Pyramid (see Chapter 3).

- Just like the Mediterranean diet guidelines, the AHA recommends eating a variety of *nutrient-dense* foods from all of the food groups, including vegetables, fruits, whole grains, legumes, and fat-free or low-fat dairy products. Some good examples are brown rice, beans, fat-free milk, and any fruit or vegetable.

- The AHA recommends eating $3\frac{1}{2}$ ounces of fish at least twice a week, much like the Mediterranean diet does.

To learn more about the guidelines of the AHA, check out their website at www.heart.org.

DEFINITION

Nutrient-dense foods contain vitamins, minerals, fiber, and other essential nutrients yet are low in calories. In other words, you get the most bang for your caloric buck with these foods. The opposite of nutrient-dense foods are empty-calorie foods, which are high in calories but low in nutritional content.

The DASH Diet

The DASH diet, which stands for Dietary Approaches to Stop Hypertension, was developed by the American Heart Association. This heart-healthy diet is meant to help people manage their high blood pressure and shares many of the same characteristics as the Mediterranean diet. The diet is easy to follow, tasty, and proven effective. It emphasizes many of the same foods that are highlighted in the Mediterranean diet: vegetables, fruits, fat-free or low-fat dairy products (it recommends a bit more dairy than what the Mediterranean diet recommends), whole grains and other high-fiber foods, fish at least twice weekly, skinless poultry, beans, seeds, and nuts. This diet plan is low in red meats, sodium, and added sugars. It focuses on consuming foods that are rich in magnesium, potassium, calcium, protein, and fiber to help lower blood pressure. Its heart-healthy label comes from the limited amounts of saturated fats, trans fats, and cholesterol that it contains. The DASH diet is about 25 to 30 percent fat.

Both the AHA Heart Healthy Guidelines and DASH diet limit fat intake a bit more than the Mediterranean diet. The Mediterranean diet focuses more on choosing your fats wisely rather than limiting them. All in all, the diets of the AHA are quite similar to the Mediterranean eating style. All are proven to be heart healthy and to decrease risk for some chronic diseases. Make room for the Mediterranean diet, because the American Heart Association's diets aren't the only reliable diets in town.

The Atkins Diet

The Atkins diet is one of the most well-known low-carbohydrate, high-protein diets around. Developed by Dr. Robert Atkins, this diet promises that you will not only lose weight but that you will also be on the road to better heart health and memory function (along with other health benefits). The Atkins diet works on the theory that people have gone "carb crazy," and that is the sole reason for the obesity problem. The diet works on the premise that consuming too many carbohydrates—especially sugar, white flour, and other refined carbs—increases insulin levels. This can lead to blood sugar imbalances, causing weight gain and other cardiovascular problems. The theory is that by eating more protein and fat and fewer carbohydrates, you will naturally lose weight by burning stored body fat more efficiently, because without the carbs, your body's main source of energy, it will use fat for energy.

The Atkins diet revolves around four phases, which don't focus on calorie counting and/or portion control, but they do require the tracking of carbs. The diet drastically restricts carbohydrates, especially in the first phase; therefore, to ensure enough calories to keep your body functioning and to make up for the lack of calories from carbohydrates, protein and fat consumption are drastically increased. Even though refined starches such as white bread, sugar, and white flours are limited, so are fruits, vegetables, whole grains, beans, and other nutritious foods that contain carbohydrates. The plan allows for protein foods that are high in saturated fats such as red meats, regular cheese, cream, butter, and more. It advocates eating a variety of fats, from unhealthy saturated fats to healthy omega-3 fatty acids. On this diet, you can eat fish and olive oil—but you can also indulge in bacon, mayonnaise, and steak with béarnaise sauce.

This diet couldn't be more contradictory to the Mediterranean diet. The Atkins diet is about restriction, while the Mediterranean diet is focused on making good choices. The Mediterranean diet is a lifestyle change, while the Atkins diet is not recommended for long-term use due to its *ketogenic* effects. Many health experts question the Atkins diet, and it remains a controversial way of eating. These types of diets are rarely successful in the long term for keeping the weight off, and they can have negative impacts on your health. Short-term effects can include headaches, muscle cramping, bad breath, diarrhea, constipation, and general fatigue. Long-term effects can include regaining weight, heart disease, certain cancers, kidney problems, diabetes complications, and osteoporosis. The Atkins theory remains unproven, unlike the benefits of the Mediterranean diet.

DEFINITION

Diets that severely restrict carbohydrates and are high in protein and fat are called **ketogenic** diets and trigger short-term weight loss through ketosis. This occurs when the body lacks enough carbohydrates, the body's main source of energy, and turns to other sources such as protein and stored fat.

The South Beach Diet

The South Beach diet was created by cardiologist Arthur Agatston, M.D. Consisting of three phases, this is another type of low-carbohydrate eating regime that touts good heart health as a result. Unlike the Atkins diet, the South Beach diet emphasizes foods that are somewhat more heart healthy by cutting out "bad" carbs, including "good" carbs, and emphasizing healthy fats. This diet is also based on the theory that people have gone "carb crazy"; however, the diet assumes that the main culprits are not *all* carbs but highly processed simple carbohydrates such as white flour and added sugars found in breads, snacks, sweets, and baked goods. The theory here is that consuming too many of these types of simple carbohydrates causes insulin resistance, which causes the body to store more fat resulting in weight gain. The diet claims that the craving for carbs disappears once you go through Phase 1 for two weeks. In addition, the diet explains that cutting out these processed, simple carbohydrates, also lowers one's triglyceride and cholesterol levels, resulting in better heart health.

Carbohydrates are basically prohibited during the initial restrictive phase of the diet and are then slowly reintroduced after two weeks. The diet stresses lean meats such as chicken, turkey, and fish as well as other protein sources, including nuts, eggs, and low-fat cheese. Once carbohydrates are reintroduced, you can have fruits, vegetables, whole grains, legumes, and others; however, you must limit consumption to keep carbohydrates at or below a specified amount. In addition, the diet relies heavily on the *glycemic index (GI)*, putting a limit on some of the foods that are allowed. There is much controversy over the GI because it is specific to individual foods. However, some factors can change the GI of foods, such as eating a certain combination of foods, how foods are cooked, and the protein and fat content. Just because a food has a high GI doesn't mean it isn't healthy—in fact, many fruits have a high GI.

> **DEFINITION**
>
> The **glycemic index (GI)** is a numerical scale that indicates how fast a single food raises blood glucose (blood sugar). The higher the GI, the quicker it will affect blood sugar. Foods that are higher in fiber or are less processed tend to have a lower GI.

The South Beach diet is similar to the Mediterranean diet in that both suggest reducing consumption of unhealthy saturated fats and promote consumption of healthy monounsaturated fats. They both emphasize "good" carbohydrates—those that are complex and less refined (such as whole grains). However, depending on which of the three phases of the South Beach diet you're in, the two diets can differ considerably. While the Mediterranean diet is high in fiber and counts on healthy, carbohydrate-containing foods as its foundation, the first phase of the South Beach diet is devoid of most of these foods. There are numerous reasons that don't make this diet as much of a lifestyle change or a way of eating for life as the Mediterranean diet.

The Ornish Diet

The Ornish diet, developed by renowned doctor Dean Ornish, is yet another alternative lifestyle approach that may help prevent, or even reverse, heart disease. Experts believe it also aids in weight loss, establishes overall good health, lowers cancer risk, and can make diabetes and hypertension more manageable. The advice in this program is supported by three decades of research. The Ornish diet not only focuses on food intake but also on other important issues such as stress reduction, exercise, and social support. Much like the Mediterranean diet, it focuses less on counting calories and more on choosing foods wisely.

Like the Mediterranean diet, the Ornish diet emphasizes lowering the intake of high-fat animal proteins such as red meats, pork, and full-fat dairy products. In addition, it is recommended to consume more complex carbohydrates such as fruits, vegetables, whole grains, and legumes as well as fat-free dairy products, egg whites, soy products, and some fish. Unlike the Mediterranean diet, it excludes meat (any type), avocados, nuts, seeds, and any oil-containing food—basically nothing with fat. This diet plan is mostly plant-based and focuses on consuming very little cholesterol or fat of any kind. Sugar and sodium are consumed very little, alcohol is prohibited, and one daily serving of soy is highly recommended.

Ornish also recommends taking supplements of omega-3 fatty acids rather than getting them from foods. If you are trying to prevent heart disease, the diet affords more discretion; however, if you are trying to reverse heart disease, it takes an even more restrictive approach.

One of the biggest differences is that the Ornish diet is extremely low in fat. This diet recommends that no more than 10 percent of calories come from fat, while the Mediterranean diet recommends a moderate fat intake of 35 to 40 percent. You can't eat much good fat (such as olive oil) on the Ornish diet if you want to stick to only 10 percent of calories from fat.

Critics say that the Ornish diet is difficult to follow and maintain due to its restrictive nature. It is said to be a healthful diet if you can live with it; however, the Mediterranean diet requires a less-drastic change in eating style to reap the health benefits.

HEALTHY MORSELS

Carbohydrates are not as bad as some diets make them out to be. In fact, carbs are an essential part of a healthy diet—the key is choosing the right ones. They provide a main source of energy, essential nutrients, and plenty of fiber. Sticking with complex carbs (such as fruits, vegetables, whole grains, and legumes) and limiting refined carbs (such as sugar and foods made with white flour) will ensure a healthy diet.

The Zone Diet

The Zone diet was developed by Dr. Barry Sears, a biochemist. The theory behind his diet again revolves around limited consumption of carbohydrates. His belief is that when you eat too many carbohydrates, a hormonal message is sent via insulin, telling the body to store fat. Dr. Sears claims that if you moderate your intake of carbohydrates and balance them with an equal proportion of fat and protein, you will enter "the zone" where you will burn fat more efficiently and revamp your metabolism, helping you to lose weight. In addition you will reduce stress, create mental clarity, improve your energy levels, and have better overall health. The Zone diet also claims that using food in this way will aid in the prevention and management of heart disease and diabetes.

What does it mean to be in "the zone"? According to Dr. Sears, it means that your meals and snacks are specifically divided:

- 40 percent of calories from carbohydrates

- 30 percent of calories from protein

- 30 percent of calories from fat

These proportions are the key to this entire diet. In addition, it's essential that meals and snacks are precisely timed: eating within 1 hour of waking up and then every 4 to 6 hours after a meal or 2 hours after a snack, even if you are not hungry. If you work the ratios and the timing the right way, the diet claims you will not be hungry and at this point you are "in the zone." Calories count in this diet plan: meals should not exceed 500 calories and snacks should be no more than 100 calories.

The Zone diet may specify certain food choices, but it doesn't leave out any food groups. Carbohydrates come mostly from fresh fruits, fresh vegetables (ones low in starch), beans, lentils, and whole grains, and protein sources include lean meats.

However, the diet specifies which carbs you can and cannot have according to their glycemic index, whether they are healthy carbs or not. Recommended fats include nuts, avocados, olive oil, and canola oil. The diet is fairly low in saturated fats. Foods high in sugar and sodium, or foods that are highly processed, are discouraged. The diet encourages drinking water and getting regular exercise. Overall the diet is much higher in protein and fat than traditional diets.

The Zone diet has received mixed reviews from nutrition experts. Some agree it includes all of the foods necessary for a healthy diet, yet others question the diet's scientific proof of its claimed health benefits. Still others feel it is just another fad diet. The American Heart Association classifies it as a high-protein diet and not optimal for weight loss.

There are some definite similarities between the Zone diet and the Mediterranean diet: both have similar food choices, both are well-balanced, and both encourage physical activity. In addition both are a bit higher in fat than traditional diets. However, there are more differences than similarities. The Zone diet can be complicated to understand and follow because it takes some work to get your fat, protein, and carbohydrate ratios exactly right at each meal and snack. This makes you wonder how easily someone could live with this type of diet for life. The Zone diet also limits carbohydrates in quantity and through the glycemic index, which differs from the Mediterranean diet that is based on these all-important foods.

The Sonoma Diet

Inspired by the Mediterranean diet, the Sonoma diet was developed by dietitian Connie Guttersen and combines the major principles of the Mediterranean diet with a typical weight-loss diet. It emphasizes eating a generous variety of healthy foods that protect your heart and boost your health. It is low in saturated fats, high in fiber, and high in heart-healthy fats.

The Sonoma diet was designed to be simple and has very little counting or measuring to complicate matters. Portion control is emphasized using the size of your plates and bowls. The diet includes phases, with the first phase being extremely restrictive. However, the diet becomes much less restrictive as you move on to the second and third phases. This diet does include foods to avoid as well as power foods to encourage.

Because this diet was designed with the Mediterranean diet in mind, there are some strong similarities—mostly with respect to the types of foods that are included. The

Sonoma diet also emphasizes eating slowly, savoring your meals, and having a glass of wine with dinner (after your initial phase, that is). However, because it is also a weight-loss diet, it has an extensive forbidden food list and very little flexibility. Even though it may seem to mimic the Mediterranean food choices, the initial phase is low in carbs and doesn't focus on as many healthy plant foods as the Mediterranean does. The biggest difference between the Mediterranean diet and the Sonoma diet is that the goal of the Sonoma diet is to lose weight, while the Mediterranean diet is more of a lifestyle change and everyday way of eating. That being said, it doesn't mean you can't lose weight by simply following the Mediterranean diet!

How to Lose Weight on the Mediterranean Diet

All of the diets we have discussed have been touted to improve heart health, though many of them are better known for their effects on weight loss. The Mediterranean diet is known first for its health benefits—especially heart health—but it can also have a positive impact on your weight. There is really no need to follow structured diets or fad diets; these are not your only means to lose weight. The Mediterranean diet certainly proves that permanent weight loss is a direct result of lifestyle change—and that is what this diet is all about.

GOOD TO KNOW

Fad diets become popular very quickly and then lose their popularity just as quickly. Many promise a quick fix, include claims that sound too good to be true, have no scientific basis, eliminate one or more of the food groups, include a must-buy product, or are not based on lifestyle changes that can help you to increase your health and lose weight permanently.

Every year people commit to new diet plans and then abandon them just as quickly because they are too restrictive either with food choices and/or calories. Many have complex phases or steps to follow and are too complicated to fit into our everyday lives. None of these describe the Mediterranean diet. It is full of wonderfully tasty and healthy foods and does not restrict you from enjoying what you like. You don't start and end your day feeling hungry and deprived. So why not use this healthy diet to your advantage?

Losing weight isn't only about the foods that you choose—there is so much more to consider. Here are some tips to make the Mediterranean diet work for your waistline as well as your health:

- Understand your true reasons for wanting to lose weight. Knowing what will motivate you and keep you committed to your goals is what will ultimately make you successful. Ponder your realistic short-term and long-term goals. Short-term goals are essential to keep you going in order to reach your long-term goals. Goals need to be specific and measurable. Write them down so you know exactly what you are working toward.

- Plan each day so that you eat three balanced meals with healthy snacks in between. Familiarize yourself with the guidelines of the Mediterranean Diet Pyramid (see Chapter 3) so that you can create a well-balanced menu. This will keep you from feeling hungry during the day and keep you from eating too much at meals or snacks. Don't skip meals!

- Plan your week's meals in advance so that you have control over what is in the house and what you eat daily. Once you've made your plan for the week, put it in writing in the form of your grocery list.

- Keep a food journal until you become comfortable with your new way of eating. Write down everything you eat, no matter how big or small. This is for your eyes only, so don't hold back. Review your journal every few days to see your progress and/or problem areas. A food journal can help you stick with the commitments you have made.

- Spend more time preparing your own meals so you know exactly what is going into the foods you are eating. The Mediterranean diet is all about fewer processed foods, so it's time to try out your culinary skills. Invest in some good cookbooks, look for recipes online, or share recipes with friends. (See Part 4 for some wonderful recipes to help get your juices flowing!)

- Read food labels when you grocery shop to choose foods that best fit into the guidelines of the Mediterranean diet. This will also give you a good measurement of portion sizes and calorie intake.

- Don't avoid your favorite foods. Deprivation can cause cravings that you just can't let go. Eat the foods you love from time to time in moderation—and watch your portion sizes.

- Do as the people of the Mediterranean do and slow down your meals and enjoy your foods. Eating too quickly can cause you to eat too much before you even realize that you're full. Eating slower can result in eating less.

- Think about the foods that you put in your mouth each and every time you eat. Make yourself accountable for what you eat and the way you live your life.

- Pay attention to portion sizes and only put small portions of food on your plate so that you are not tempted to overeat. Use a smaller plate if you need to. Portion your food out before bringing your plate to the table and refrain from eating while doing other tasks like watching television or working at the computer.

- Experiment with new foods and fill your plate with a rainbow of colors. The more colors you have on your plate, the more nutrition you have in your meal. The Mediterranean diet is full of a variety of tasty foods—use that to your advantage.

- Follow the guidelines of the Mediterranean diet for all foods but especially for fruits, vegetables, whole grains, beans, and lentils. These foods are packed with fiber, which can be very filling and help you to eat fewer calories.

- Drink plenty of water throughout each day. Staying properly hydrated is essential to digestion and the fat-burning process. It can also help you with portion control at meals or with snacks.

- Be physically active each and every day. Obesity is a direct result of an imbalance between the calories you take in and the calories you burn—it's just that simple. The more active you are, the more calories you will burn. Something as simple as walking can be a great start.

These simple tips and changes can help you to improve your health and reduce your waistline on the Mediterranean diet. Remember that it is all about lifestyle changes that you can stick with. Losing weight slowly over time is more manageable and, experts agree, more permanent. Make changes to both your eating style and your lifestyle a little at a time—and most importantly, stick with your commitment to become a healthier person.

The Least You Need to Know

- Experts agree that the Mediterranean diet is indeed a preferred way of life.
- The Mediterranean diet favorably compares with the American Heart Association's recommendations and the DASH diet.
- The Mediterranean diet comes out on top compared to many of the diets that claim to be heart healthy.
- You can lose weight on the Mediterranean diet with the right motivation, commitment, and helpful tips.

Transitioning Your Diet

In This Chapter

- Looking at your foods differently
- The foods included on the Mediterranean diet
- Satisfying your sweet tooth
- Understanding what's on the food label
- The Mediterranean Food Alliance and Med Mark

Transitioning your current diet to the Mediterranean style of eating is a smart way to begin taking control of your health. Some aspects might be easier than others but the key is to transition slowly. Don't be determined to change everything all at once. Make changes to your diet and lifestyle habits one step at a time—before you know it, you will be transitioned to the Mediterranean way of life and reaping all of the health benefits. It's time to take action!

Foods to Reduce and Foods to Add

As always, moderation is the key. Begin to reduce or replace the foods in your diet gradually. If your current diet needs a lot of help, the last thing you want to do is jump in with both feet. Instead, start slowly but progress steadily by gradually reducing the foods you don't need and replacing them with the foods you do. The Mediterranean diet is not one of deprivation but rather one that is jam-packed with a variety of healthy foods, so adding foods should be painless.

Foods to reduce:

- Start by reducing portions of the foods in your diet that are not part of the Mediterranean diet. That includes red meats, whole-fat dairy products, fried foods, fast foods, and high-calorie sweets. Continue to reduce them until you have eliminated them.

- Replace portions of your foods with food from the Mediterranean. For example, if you are going to cook with ground beef, replace half with ground turkey breast.

- Trade your full-fat dairy products for low-fat or, better yet, fat-free products. Choose low-fat or nonfat yogurt and cheeses. Not quite at the point of drinking fat-free milk? Start by mixing equal amounts of fat-free and 2 percent milk.

- Prepare to eat fewer fatty foods such as animal products, especially red meat. This is eaten very rarely in the Mediterranean diet and one of the first foods you need to begin reducing to make a successful transition. Start by reducing it to once or twice a week and transition down to a few times a month, if that.

- Think fresh and begin to reduce your consumption of processed foods. There is no room in the Mediterranean diet for white sugar, white flour, junk foods, and other foods that come neatly packaged and processed. Shopping the outside aisles of the grocery store will ensure you are choosing fresher foods.

- Reduce your use of butter and/or margarine in cooking and preparing foods until you have completely replaced it with healthier fats such as olive oil over time.

Foods to add:

- Load up on fresh fruits and vegetables wherever possible. In addition, cook with them by trying out new recipes. Your daily diet should be packed with these foods as they make up a good proportion of the Mediterranean diet.

- Start to think of your grains in a different way. Begin steering away from the refined grains you might be used to such as white breads, white rice, and regular pasta and turn to whole grains such as oatmeal, whole-grain bread, brown rice, whole-wheat pasta, bulgur, and couscous.

- Use olive oil for cooking, as a replacement for butter or margarine on breads and vegetables, and as a salad dressing. Olive oil is the backbone of the Mediterranean diet.

- Rely on leaner protein choices, such as fish and skinless white meat chicken or turkey, to replace your red meat. Include fish a few times in your weekly meal plans.

- Add a few meatless meals to your weekly meal plans. This will help you to cut back on red meat and other saturated fats. Meat isn't the only way to get the protein you need at meals. Try basing some meals on beans, legumes, low-fat cheeses, and nuts.

Changing Your Approach

Adopting a new lifestyle means changing how you think about different foods and habits. You need to move away from old habits and adopt new ones, and that can take some work. You have to think as the people of the Mediterranean would and approach what you would normally eat with a new attitude.

TO YOUR HEALTH

Sandwiches are not as popular in the Mediterranean as they are in the United States—so how do you update your sandwich to give it some Mediterranean flair? Instead of two pieces of white bread filled with high-fat deli meat, full-fat cheese, and mayonnaise, consider a vegetable sandwich: red peppers, eggplant, tomatoes, mushrooms, and/or zucchini topped with low-fat cheese and a touch of olive oil stuffed into a whole-wheat pita. If you like, add a few chunks of white meat chicken or broiled fish. You can even add a bit of brown rice. You've just changed your approach to sandwiches!

Changing your approach to food isn't as hard as you might think. Take pasta, for example. In the typical Western diet, we might cover pasta with meaty spaghetti sauce or a creamy Alfredo sauce, both loaded with unhealthy fats. To make it Mediterranean, you could simply use whole-grain pasta and toss it with fresh-cut tomatoes, garlic, fresh basil, and olive oil. You could even throw in some fresh spinach, mushrooms, and peas to make it a filling, healthy meal.

The possibilities are endless. It takes a new thought process on your end to take the foods you normally eat and find a way to fit them into the Mediterranean diet. That goes not only for the meals and snacks but also for lifestyle habits like exercise and drinking.

Essential Food List of the Mediterranean Diet

There is a huge variety of foods that are included on the Mediterranean diet. Remember, it is not a diet of deprivation but one of healthy choices. These might be foods that you have never tried or foods that you already incorporate into your own diet. If your pantry is stocked with the foods you need to follow the Mediterranean diet, it will be easier for you to plan and prepare meals on a regular basis.

See the applicable chapter (Chapter 8 on fruits, for example) for much more information about a food group.

Breads, Grains, and Pastas

Brown rice
Couscous
Oatmeal
Polenta
Quinoa
Rye bread
Wheat berries
Whole-grain bread
Whole-grain pita bread
Whole-wheat pasta (any kind)

Flours

Barley
Buckwheat
Bulgur
Farro (spelt)
Unbleached all-purpose
Whole-wheat

Dairy Products

Asiago cheese
Cottage cheese (low-fat)
Feta cheese
Goat cheese
Mozzarella cheese
Provolone cheese
Ricotta cheese
Milk (fat-free or low-fat)
Yogurt (plain or fruited, fat-free or
  low-fat; Greek)

Fruits

Apricots
Avocados
Blueberries
Cherries
Dates
Dried fruit

Fruits (continued)

Figs
Melon (cantaloupe/honeydew)
Olives
Pomegranates
Strawberries

Legumes

Black beans
Black-eyed peas
Borlotti beans (cranberry beans)
Cannellini beans (white kidney beans)
Chickpeas (garbanzo beans)
Fava beans (broad beans)
Lentils
Pinto beans
Split peas

Meats

Chicken, white meat, skinless
Ground beef, lean
Lamb
Turkey, white meat, skinless
Turkey, breast, ground
Veal

Miscellaneous

Eggs
Honey
Hummus
Phyllo dough
Spices such as basil, garlic, mint,
  oregano, paprika, and rosemary
Tahini
Tomato paste
Balsamic vinegar
Wine vinegar

Nuts and Seeds

Almonds
Cashews
Chestnuts
Flaxseeds
Hazelnuts
Peanuts
Pine nuts
Pistachios
Sesame seeds
Sunflower seeds
Walnuts

Oils

Canola
Grapeseed
Olive oil, extra-virgin

Seafood/Fish

Clams
Crab
Halibut
Octopus
Salmon
Sardines
Shrimp
Squid
Swordfish
Tilapia
Tuna

Vegetables

Arugula
Artichoke hearts
Bell pepper (red/green)
Broccoli
Cabbage
Celery, celery leaves, celery root

Vegetables (continued)

Dandelion greens

Eggplant

Grape leaves

Mushrooms

Mustard greens

Onions

Pepperoncinis

Spinach

Swiss chard

Tomatoes, fresh, canned, sun-dried

Zucchini

What About Sweets?

Because the majority of us have a sweet tooth, transitioning to the Mediterranean diet, where sweets are eaten only a few times a week and in small amounts, can be a big change. Desserts are more of an afterthought as opposed to an expected ending to a meal. Sometimes sweets accompany afternoon tea or coffee. In the Mediterranean, what follows a meal leans more towards fresh fruits and nuts instead of sweets with added sugar and fat. Fruit can be fresh, baked, stewed, or cooked into jams or tarts. A fruity dessert makes the perfect end to a healthy meal. Check out the yummy dessert recipes in Chapter 22.

How can you change your approach to the way you think about sweets? The Mediterranean diet embraces naturally sweetened foods rather than added sugar. Honey is commonly used as the natural sweetener in many Mediterranean meals and desserts. It's widely used to sweeten plain yogurt and in place of sugar in coffee or tea. It makes a nice addition to toast and breads, and you can even drizzle it on your salad along with a little olive oil, lemon, and vinegar.

Honey isn't just another sweetener. Did you know that honey can actually be beneficial to your health and even help to boost your immune system? This natural sweetener contains vitamins, minerals, antioxidants, enzymes, and even a few amino acids (the building blocks of protein). Honey's antibacterial and antioxidant properties can help aid in digestion, help to keep you healthy, and fight disease. There is a wide assortment of floral honey varieties—23 to be exact—all with unique flavors of their own. Leave it to the people of the Mediterranean to find a way to enjoy something sweet that is also good for you!

HEALTHY MORSELS

Honey contains about 64 calories per tablespoon while refined table sugar contains about 46 calories per tablespoon. However, because honey is much sweeter than table sugar, you can use less of it. As a result, you may consume fewer calories using honey versus table sugar. In addition, table sugar—unlike honey—is empty calories, meaning it contains no nutritional value.

Reading the Food Label

The Mediterranean diet is all about choosing healthier foods. We can all use a little help when trying to pick out healthier foods, and that's where the Nutrition Facts Panel on food labels can help out. People of the Mediterranean consume mostly fresh foods—in that area of the world, it is much more realistic—but we may need a little extra help weeding through the foods available at our local supermarkets. Food labels will help you to uncover nutrition facts about the foods you buy. Learning and understanding the differences in the types of fats and knowing how to interpret other parts of the food label can help you to become a much smarter food shopper and more equipped to choose foods that fit into the Mediterranean way of life.

The Nutrition Facts Panel

What we are specifically referring to on a packaged food's label is termed the Nutrition Facts Panel. This panel is full of detailed nutrition information. It includes nutrients that people often consume in excess and that should be limited because they can increase the risk for chronic diseases. These nutrients include total fat, saturated fat, trans fat, cholesterol, and sodium. Other nutrients are listed because they often come up short in the typical diet and eating enough of these nutrients can help to improve health and lower risk for some chronic health conditions. These nutrients include dietary fiber, vitamin A, vitamin C, calcium, and iron. Other nutrients listed include total carbohydrates, sugar (including both naturally occurring and added sugars), and protein. Some manufacturers may include additional nutrients, but those mentioned previously are required. The information on the panel is important enough that it is required by the FDA (Food and Drug Administration) and USDA on most packaged foods. Food labels also include other helpful information, including an ingredient list and optional health and nutrient content claims. All of this information is there to help consumers make healthier food choices.

The key place to start when reading the Nutrition Facts Panel is right from the top. That is because the first listing is the serving size, and all of the information on the panel pertains to that all-important serving size. Serving sizes on packaged foods are standardized to make it easier for consumers to compare nutritional facts on similar foods. For example, the standard serving size on salad dressing, no matter what the brand name, is two tablespoons. That makes it easier to pick up two bottles of dressing and carefully compare their nutritional content. You can also find servings per container at the top of the panel. Be careful not to fall into the trap of assuming there is only one serving in a package. All of the information on the label pertains to *one* serving—so if it states there are two servings per package, you need to double all of the numbers if you plan to eat the whole thing!

TO YOUR HEALTH

As a general guide to calories, 40 to 99 calories per single serving of a food is considered low, 100 to 399 calories is considered moderate, and 400 calories or more is considered high. This universal guide provides a general reference and is based on an average 2,000-calorie diet. Eating too many high-calorie foods on a daily basis can cause you to take in more calories than your body needs, which can be directly linked to obesity-related health problems. By reading the food label and being aware of calories you can balance your daily calories and better manage your weight.

Check Out the Label's Nutrients

All of the nutrients listed on the Nutrition Facts Panel are important; however, when it comes to the Mediterranean diet, some are more crucial than others at helping you to stick with your new way of eating:

- **Fat.** Look at not only total fat, but also what makes up that fat. Is it mostly saturated fats and trans fats or is it mostly healthy fats of the Mediterranean diet (such as monounsaturated fat)?

- **Sodium.** Be sure to check the sodium content, because the Mediterranean diet is low in this nutrient.

- **Fiber.** Not only do you get this essential nutrient from fruits and vegetables but also in whole grains like breads, beans, rice, cereals, and pasta, so check the panel for the amount of fiber the product is supplying.

- **Sugar.** The Mediterranean diet has a low sugar content, so check out how much of the carbohydrate is made up of sugar.

Let's not forget the ingredient list, which can clue you in to other nutritional dilemmas. Ingredient lists are required on food labels for any food that contains more than one ingredient. Ingredient lists must be listed in descending order by weight. If you take a look at a cereal box, for example, and sugar is the first ingredient listed, don't buy it. There are ingredients that you should limit or avoid when eating a healthier diet. For instance, if a food has less than 0.5 grams of trans fat per serving, it can be listed as zero on the Nutrition Facts Panel, but hydrogenated or partially hydrogenated oils will be listed in the ingredient list. This will clue you in to whether a food contains trans fat, an unhealthy, artery-clogging fat. Although 0.5 grams of trans fat seems small, you could exceed recommended amounts if you eat multiple servings of that food.

TO YOUR HEALTH

For heart health, choose foods with a lower combined total of saturated fat plus trans fat plus a lower amount of cholesterol.

Percent Daily Value

Not sure if a serving of food has a little or a lot of a particular nutrient? That is where the Percent Daily Value (%DV) comes in. You will find the %DV on the right side of the panel for most of the nutrients. This percentage is an average of how a single serving of a particular food meets the daily requirements for each nutrient, based on a 2,000-calorie diet. It is important to remember that %DV refers to what you need for the entire day, not in a single meal or snack. Depending on your individual calorie needs, you may need more or less than 2,000 calories per day—so for some nutrients you may need more or less than what is listed as 100 percent of the DV. But the %DV will provide you with a frame of reference to decide whether or not the food will provide an appropriate amount of a specific nutrient, and it can help you determine if a serving of food is high or low in a specific nutrient:

- **5 percent or less DV is low.** Aim for this amount for all nutrients that you want to limit in your diet.

- **10 to 19 percent DV is moderate.** This indicates that the food is a good source for the nutrients you want to consume in greater amounts.

- **20 percent or more DV is high.** This indicates that the food is an excellent source for nutrients you want to consume in greater amounts.

You don't need to know how to calculate the %DV because the label does that for you. At the bottom of the Nutrition Facts Panel, you will find the Reference Daily Values that are used to calculate the percentages. These values, like everything on the panel, are based on an average daily intake of 2,000 calories.

HEALTHY MORSELS

There are several nutrients listed on the label that do not require %DV. These include trans fats, protein, and sugar. Trans fats do not yet have sufficient data to establish a Daily Value. Protein only needs a %DV if the food claims to be high in protein or if it's to be used for children under four years of age, because protein is not indicated as a health concern. Sugar has no %DV because no recommendations have been made for the total amount you should eat in a day.

There are many reasons to use the Nutrition Facts Panel on food labels. If you plan to follow a Mediterranean diet, it can be very helpful in choosing the right foods. Reading the panel can take some practice, but once you have mastered use of the label, it can come in very handy. Be sure to scan the entire label and look at the whole food as opposed to only looking for one nutrient. For example, a food can be low in fat but not hold any other nutritional value, or it can be fat-free but loaded with sugar and/or sodium.

Be Aware of Health and Nutrient Content Claims

Health and nutrient content claims can also appear on a food label. Both types of claims are strictly defined and regulated by the FDA and can help you to easily find foods that meet your specific nutrition goals.

Nutrient content claims such as *low fat* or *high fiber* can make it easy to find foods that will help you reach your goals. Following the Mediterranean diet, you might look for claims that deal with fat, fiber, sodium, sugar, and cholesterol. These nutrient content claims usually show up on the front of the food's label or package for quick information. They pertain to a single serving and are an optional part of the label. An example might be the label term *free*, as in fat-free, calorie-free, or sodium-free. In these examples, *free* means the amount of fat, calories, or sodium in one serving of the food is so small that it probably won't have an effect on your body. There are also regulated definitions for *low, reduced, high, good source, more, light, healthy,* and, on meat, *lean* and *extra lean*.

GOOD TO KNOW

Just because a food is labeled *cholesterol-free* doesn't necessarily mean that it is healthy and will fit into the Mediterranean diet. Some foods contain hydrogenated or partially hydrogenated oils, which are trans fats. The same goes for foods labeled *sodium-free*, which could contain high amounts of sugar and, therefore, empty calories. Always check the Nutrition Facts Panel to get the whole story—even if a claim is included on the packaging.

Health claims link a food, or components of a food, with a decreased risk for some chronic disease. As with nutrient content claims, health claims will show up on the front of a food's label or packaging. These claims are optional and yet highly regulated. Only certain health claims have been approved on foods and these claims are supported by strong scientific evidence. Some of the health claims that might be of particular interest for the Mediterranean diet include:

- To make health claims about sodium and hypertension, a food must be low in sodium.

- To make health claims about dietary fat and cancer, a food must be low in fat or fat-free.

- To make health claims about heart disease, a food must be low in fat, saturated fat, and cholesterol.

- To make health claims about fiber-containing grain products, fruits, and vegetables and cancer, a food must be a good source of fiber and low in fat.

- To make health claims about fruits, vegetables, and grain products that contain fiber, particularly soluble fiber, and their risk of coronary heart disease, a food must be low in fat, saturated fat, and cholesterol, as well as have at least 0.6 grams of soluble fiber (without fortification) per serving and list soluble fiber on the label.

- To make health claims about fruits and vegetables and cancer, a food must be low in fat and a good source (without fortification) of vitamin A, vitamin C, or fiber.

Look for foods with these health claims and you are bound to find a food that will fit well into your Mediterranean eating plan.

All About the Mediterranean Foods Alliance and Med Mark

The Mediterranean Foods Alliance (MFA) was created by the Oldways Preservation & Exchange Trust to help consumers more easily incorporate foods of the Mediterranean diet into their daily meal plans. They found that even though people heard about the wonderful benefits of the Mediterranean diet and wanted to eat in the Mediterranean style, they weren't always sure how to incorporate it into their everyday lives—or into their shopping carts at the grocery store. The MFA was created to be a one-stop consumer education program to help guide people on how to shop for, prepare, and enjoy healthy foods that fit into the Mediterranean way of life. The MFA is meant to be a resource for consumers, chefs, retailers, health professionals, journalists—anyone who wants to better understand and incorporate the Mediterranean diet.

As a result of the MFA, the Med Mark was developed. The Med Mark is an easily recognizable symbol used on qualifying product packages that meet the MFA's strict nutrition criteria. The Med Mark packaging symbol is meant to help consumers find healthy Mediterranean diet products in their favorite grocery stores. This simple symbol lets you know that the foods and drinks you are choosing are considered to be a core part of the Mediterranean diet.

At present there are about 150 food products that bear the Med Mark symbol. Not only do these foods meet the nutrition criteria of the Mediterranean diet, but they are also consistent with the FDA's definition of healthy (a food low in fat, saturated fat, cholesterol, and sodium and contains at least 10 percent of the Daily Values for vitamin A, vitamin C, iron, calcium, protein, and fiber).

For foods to be eligible to use the Med Mark, processed foods or food products not sold in their natural, minimally processed state must meet the following criteria (per serving):

- The product must contain no added trans fats in any amount (limit of 0 grams).

- The product must contain no more than 8 percent of total calories from saturated fat.

- The product must contain no more than 480 mg of sodium for side items and snacks and no more than 600 mg for meals.

- The product must contain no more than 4 grams of added sugar (about 1 teaspoon).

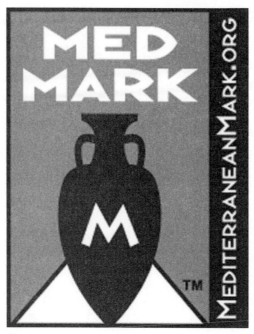

The Med Mark symbol.
Courtesy Oldways and the Mediterranean Foods Alliance; www.oldwayspt.org and
www.mediterraneanmark.org.

As more foods become eligible for the Med Mark, the easier it will become to choose
the foods you need to follow the Mediterranean diet. For more information and a list
of foods currently allowing the Med Mark symbol, go to www.mediterraneanmark.
org.

The Least You Need to Know

- Become familiar with the foods you need to begin adding and reducing to
  begin the gradual transition to a Mediterranean lifestyle.
- Honey is a way to naturally sweeten foods and can also be good for your health.
- Reviewing the Nutrition Facts Panel can help you make better food choices for a
  healthy diet.
- The Med Mark symbol is an invaluable tool that can help you to easily choose
  foods specific to the Mediterranean diet.

Olive Oil 101

In This Chapter

- The story of olive oil
- Olive oil and the Mediterranean diet
- Why all the hype about olive oil?
- Making the best choice
- Shelf life and storage
- Cooking and baking with olive oil

Olive oil has been around for a long time, yet experts are still discovering additional health benefits and new ways to use it. Olive oil is the only oil that can be used as is, freshly pressed and minimally processed from the olive itself. Best of all, olive oil is free of cholesterol, sodium, trans fat, and sugar, and is a rich and healthy source of monounsaturated fats and other essential nutrients, including antioxidants and phytonutrients.

The History and Making of Olive Oil

Olive oil comes from olives, which are grown on trees that originate from the regions of the Mediterranean basin. There is a history of over 6,000 years of olive tree cultivation in these regions. At one time the oil from olives was used not only for food but also for beauty treatments, fuel for oil lamps, medicinal purposes, and even soap making. Currently, olive oil continues to grow in popularity and usage—it is becoming big business as its health benefits are becoming well documented. It plays a part not only in Mediterranean cuisine but also in cuisines all over the world, even in the Western culture of today.

Turning olives into oil is a delicate process. Olive oil is obtained from the pressing and centrifuging of crushed olives. However, there are different techniques for the pressing or extraction process, and each individual grower will have their own unique method. The way in which the olives are picked, shipped, handled, and pressed all play a role in the ultimate quality and grade of the oil.

HEALTHY MORSELS

Olives are actually a fruit—hence the reason olive oil is put into the plant group of the Mediterranean Diet Pyramid.

You might find extraction methods described on olive oil labels. Cold extraction processes retain more nutrients as well as color, flavor, and the aroma of olives. Heat extraction processes can take a toll on delicate olives and will destroy much of the fragile nutrients with just about all of the color, flavor, and aroma.

There are varieties of olive oil from all over the globe. Most of the worldwide supply is produced from olives grown in Greece, Spain, and Italy. Spain supplies about 45 percent of the world's olive supply. This oil is usually golden yellow–colored oil with a fruity, nutty flavor. Italian olive oil is often dark green with an herbal aroma. Italy is responsible for about 20 percent of the world's olives. Greek olive oil is generally highly flavored and aromatic. Greece grows about 13 percent of the world's olive supply. Other areas, including California, Australia, and France, have begun producing olive oil as well. Olive oil from France and California tends to be milder in flavor and lighter in color. Olive oil from Australia is mostly exported to Asia and Europe. The oil's flavor can vary quite a bit depending on where the olives were grown and whether the oil was produced from olives from a single region or as a blend of olives from several regions. If you try a particular brand and don't like the flavor, simply try another until you find the one that suits your taste.

Connection to the Mediterranean Diet

Olive oil is essentially the backbone of the Mediterranean diet, at least partly due to the simple fact that olive trees are abundant in the Mediterranean. With all its amazing health benefits, it remains the principal fat source in the Mediterranean region and a daily staple in many Mediterranean homes. Olive oil complements the traditional flavors and dishes of the Mediterranean cuisine. It's not the only food that creates this diet's health benefits, but it is a major component.

A Daily Occurrence

Olive oil is used abundantly in cooking, baking, marinating, and dressings through-out the Mediterranean. It is one of the foods that contributes to the diet's high proportion of heart-healthy monounsaturated fats. To reap the health benefits of this healthy oil and to follow the guidelines of the Mediterranean diet, olive oil should be a part of your everyday diet.

Can't figure out how to get more olive oil into your diet? Here are some tips:

- Use olive oil instead of dressing on your salads. Add a bit of red wine vinegar and lemon as well.

- Dip your 100 percent whole-grain bread in olive oil and do away with the butter or margarine. Add a bit of oregano, black pepper, or Parmesan cheese for added flavor.

- Sprinkle freshly cooked vegetables with olive oil, including baked potatoes and corn on the cob.

- Scramble your eggs or cook your omelets in olive oil instead of butter or margarine.

- Toss it into your favorite pasta with fresh veggies.

- Brush the bread for grilled sandwiches with olive oil instead of margarine or butter.

- Use olive oil to baste meat or seafood before and during grilling and roasting.

- Use olive oil in recipes in place of vegetable oils or other fats.

- Use olive oil, along with herbs and spices, to marinate meats, seafood, or vegetables before cooking.

- Use olive oil to prepare spreads or dips such as hummus.

- Stir-fry lean meat or seafood and your favorite vegetables in olive oil.

Healthy Benefits

Olive oil is a fat, but don't let the word *fat* fool you—its high content of healthy monounsaturated fats makes olive oil quite healthy. Studies have consistently shown that one of the key benefits to consuming olive oil is that it helps lower cholesterol.

It is the monounsaturated fats that help to lower the bad cholesterol (or LDL) and increase the good cholesterol (or HDL), and both of these are important factors for good heart health. The key to getting the health benefits from this oil is not just to add olive oil to your current diet but to use it as a replacement for unhealthy fats, the way the Mediterranean diet does.

With the discovery of all the health benefits of olive oil, the FDA released a qualified health claim in 2004 linking monounsaturated fatty acids from olive oil with reduced risk of coronary heart disease. Olive oil and olive oil–containing products may list the following claim on their labels or in their advertising: "Limited and not conclusive scientific evidence suggests that eating about 2 tablespoons (23 grams) of olive oil daily may reduce the risk of coronary heart disease due to the monounsaturated fat in olive oil. To achieve this possible benefit, olive oil is to replace a similar amount of saturated fat and not increase the total number of calories you eat in a day. One serving of this product contains x grams of olive oil." (Note: the last sentence is optional when the claim is used on the label or in the labeling of olive oil.)

With all the research being done on this wonderful oil, researchers are finding even more health benefits. The rich supplies of polyphenols in olive oil, which are not found in many nut and seed oils, are natural antioxidants and have been shown to have anti-inflammatory and anticoagulant properties. This is central to evidence that olive oil can lower cholesterol, blood pressure, and the risk for heart disease as well as protect against certain cancers and even osteoporosis.

Olive oil is well tolerated by the stomach and it may also have a protective function against ulcers, gastritis, and gallstones. In addition, the omega-3 fatty acids in olive oil help keep blood cells from sticking together, increase blood flow, and help to reduce inflammation, making these fats useful not only for preventing cardiovascular disease but also inflammatory conditions such as arthritis. Because of the antioxidants, phytonutrients, and healthy fats that olive oil contains, it may also help to slow down the process of aging and the many chronic conditions that follow.

TO YOUR HEALTH

When picking out olive oil, choose one with a green or yellow tint. These oils come from ripe olives and may contain more polyphenols, a powerful antioxidant that can benefit the heart.

Nutritional Properties of Olive Oil

Olive oil is considered a monounsaturated fat. As with other oils, it is made up of more than one type of fat, but it is predominantly comprised of monounsaturated fatty acids (or oleic acids). In fact, no other naturally produced oil has such a large monounsaturated fat content. From a nutritional standpoint, the fat content in a typical olive oil averages about:

- 75 percent oleic acid (an omega-9 monounsaturated fat)
- 10 percent linoleic acid (an omega-6 polyunsaturated fat)
- 1 percent linolenic acid (an omega-3 polyunsaturated fat)
- 15 percent saturated fat

The U.S. Dietary Reference Intakes for essential fatty acids currently recommends consuming omega-6 and omega-3 fats in a ratio of 10 to 1. It is amazing how nature provides that exact ratio in olive oil.

Fat isn't the only component that makes up olive oil. This oil is rich in essential vitamins and antioxidants such as thiamin, riboflavin, niacin, and vitamins A, C, E, and K. You can even find a bit of iron and other essential nutrients. In addition, it's full of polyphenols and flavonoids, both of which are powerful phytonutrients and health promoters.

Olive oil outweighs other fats when it comes to its content of health-promoting monounsaturated fats. Even fats that contain decent amounts of monounsaturated fats contain way too much saturated fat. Look for yourself and compare!

A Comparison of Fats

Type of Fat	Monounsaturated	Polyunsaturated	Saturated
Olive oil	75%	10%	15%
Canola oil	62%	31%	7%
Peanut oil	48%	33%	19%
Palm oil	39%	9%	52%
Butter	30%	5%	65%
Corn oil	25%	62%	13%
Soybean oil	25%	60%	15%

continues

A Comparison of Fats (continued)

Type of Fat	Monounsaturated	Polyunsaturated	Saturated
Sunflower oil	21%	68%	11%
Flaxseed oil	18%	73%	9%
Coconut oil	6%	2%	92%

GOOD TO KNOW

Olive oil is full of health benefits, but don't overdo it. Remember to consume olive oil in moderation (2 tablespoons daily) as it has 120 calories per tablespoon.

Sorting Out the Varieties

Choosing an olive oil can be mind-boggling without the right information. There are different grades of olive oil; some are more flavorful and provide more health benefits than others. Olive oil is graded on taste, acidity level, and processing method. Certain types of olive oils are better for certain cooking methods and recipes. The many variables that go into producing olive oil such as the variety of olive, where the olive is grown, ripeness when picked, time of harvesting, pressing technique, packaging, and storage can all generate remarkable differences in color, aroma, and flavor. Each type of olive oil carries its own classification, which is used to differentiate between all of the varieties.

Extra-Virgin Olive Oil

At the head of the class sits the extra-virgin olive oil varieties. These can include label classifications such as *premium extra-virgin* and *extra-virgin* oils. These are the highest-quality olive oils made from the first pressing of the olives with no heat or chemicals and very low levels of acidity (no more than 0.8 percent). Acidity levels correspond with the type of olives used as well as with storage and production methods. A low acidity level is a key factor when choosing a great-tasting, high-quality olive oil. Extra-virgin olive oil has the lowest acidity level, but as it gets older the acidity can rise a little and change the flavor slightly. These oils are unrefined and contain higher levels of antioxidants, particularly vitamin E and polyphenols, because it is less processed. For your health's sake, this is the best choice.

A wide range of flavors can be found in extra-virgin olive oils. Flavor is determined by many factors, including the type and ripeness of olive used, growing conditions, harvesting methods, storage, and pressing methods. In general, the deeper the color, the more flavor the oil will yield. The color of these high-quality oils should be a deep greenish-gold color. Extra-virgin olive oil is great for dipping bread; as a dressing or marinade; and for drizzling over vegetables, stews, or fish. The highest-quality extra-virgin olive oils have a buttery taste and can be used to replace other fats, such as butter or margarine, on breads. Because heat can change both its flavor and nutritional content, extra-virgin olive oil is best used in uncooked dishes or as a finishing touch in order to properly appreciate its excellent aroma and flavor.

HEALTHY MORSELS

If you are looking for a high-quality extra-virgin olive oil, look for bottles that are certified by the International Olive Oil Council (IOOC). The IOOC standard oils must meet certain criteria before being placed into a specific category. These olive oils cannot be combined with any other type of oil and they must pass through a certified panel of tasters, meet analytical criteria, and prove genuineness and purity.

Virgin Olive Oil

Next in line is virgin olive oil. These oils can include label classifications such as *fine virgin* and *semifine virgin*. Virgin olive oil, like extra-virgin olive oil, is made from the first pressing of the olives. It is made with no chemicals or high heat and is unrefined. The difference between the two oils and their grade is around a percentage point of acidity. However, in the world of olive oils, that's all it takes to distinguish between very good oils and great oils. Virgin olive oil is great for salad dressings and marinades and also works well in uncooked dishes. The taste is not quite as pronounced as extra-virgin olive oil, but it still has a good flavor.

Fine virgin olive oil must have a good flavor by industry standards and an acidity level of no more than 1.5 percent. This oil is less expensive than the extra-virgin olive oil, but is very close in quality. Virgin olive oil must also have a good flavor, but the acidity can be no more than 2 percent. This oil is good for cooking, but it also has enough flavor to enjoy it uncooked. Semifine virgin olive oil must have an acidity level no higher than 3.3 percent. It is best used for cooking as the flavor isn't strong enough to be enjoyed in uncooked dishes.

Olive Oil

One more step down the ladder you will find olive oil that can be labeled as *pure olive oil* or *refined oil*. Pure olive oil consists of a blend of both refined olive oil and virgin olive oil. Refined olive oil is obtained from virgin olive oil by refining methods. Refining refers to oils that have been chemically treated, using charcoal and other chemical and physical filters, to neutralize strong tastes as well as acid content. Oils that are further refined after the first pressing can no longer carry the title *virgin*. These oils carry a much milder flavor and are good for sautéing, where virgin oils are not due to their low *smoke point*. These oils are also ideal for basting, grilling, and a good choice for pasta dishes.

DEFINITION

The **smoke point** of oil is the temperature at which the oil will smoke when heated. If an oil is heated past its smoke point, it is no longer good for use or good for you. Refined olive oils have a slightly higher smoke point (about 410°F) then nonrefined olive oils (400°F).

Lite Olive Oil

The word *lite* refers to oils that have been refined. Lite olive oil is also called *light* or *mild* oil. These words don't mean that the oil is lower in fat or calories but rather refers to its light or mild flavor. These oils are highly refined or processed to extract the last bit of possible oil from the olives. These oils contain the same amount of healthy monounsaturated fats as all of the other olive oils, but much of the color, aroma, and flavor is lost due to the refining process. Other nutritional content is also lost, such as vitamins and antioxidants. These are more suitable for cooking or baking and in recipes where strong flavor is not desired. The refining process also gives these oils a higher smoke point, making them a better candidate for high-heat cooking methods.

Handle with Care

Now you know olive oil will be a staple in your pantry. But how long should it stay there? How should it be stored? Oils can be fragile and need to be handled with care. The four enemies of olive oil are age, heat, air, and light. Restricting all of these will greatly extend its shelf life and keep it from turning rancid, which would destroy all the healthy antioxidant properties of the oil.

Because heat, air, and light do so much damage to olive oil, your best bet is to keep it in a dark, cool cupboard. Tinted glass bottles or stainless steel make optimal containers. Avoid other metals such as iron or copper, which when in contact with olive oil can create toxic compounds. Also avoid the use of most plastics, because oil can leach out toxic compounds from the plastic. The cap or lid on the container needs to be tight to keep out unwanted air. Storage temperature is important—room temperature, about 70 degrees, will do just fine. Keep the oil out of cupboards that are near your oven or other heat sources. If your kitchen seems to be too warm most of the time, try refrigerating your oil. You can keep small amounts at room temperature for daily use and put the remainder in the refrigerator. Keep in mind that refrigerated olive oil will solidify and turn cloudy until returned to room temperature.

GOOD TO KNOW

Oil experts don't recommend storing premium extra-virgin olive oils in the refrigerator because condensation can develop and affect flavor. Your best bet for these oils is room temperature. Other olive oils do fine with refrigeration.

Because of olive oil's high content of monounsaturated fat, it can be stored longer than other oils if stored properly. In fact, high-quality olive oils will retain their quality and flavor for at least a year, while lower-quality olive oils will last only a few months. Unopened, olive oil will keep for as long as two years. Olive oil doesn't get better with age; in fact, as it ages, acidity rises, flavor diminishes, and nutritional content decreases. Extra-virgin olive oils keep a bit longer because it starts with a lower acidity level. Not all bottles carry bottling dates or "use by" dates but it's worth checking if the bottle does have one before you buy. Don't let your olive oil just sit in the cupboard—use it up!

Bright light can be a destroyer of oil. In some grocery stores, especially ones open 24 hours, bottles of olive oil can have bright light beating on them all day long. Look for bottles that are not stored on the top shelf or in front. Instead, grab a bottle from the second row where direct light isn't reaching it. Also, look for brands that come in a dark-colored bottle. If you are grabbing from the very back, make sure the bottle is free of dust, which might signify it has been sitting on the shelf for quite some time.

Cooking with Olive Oil

Cooking with olive oil is a great way to include its health benefits in your daily diet. Olive oil helps to bring out the natural flavor of foods, herbs, and spices. The extra-virgin and virgin varieties are your best choices to use uncooked or cooked at a low to medium temperature. Refined olive oil and olive oil grades are better choices for high heat such as sautéing. Smoke point is important; an oil's smoke point is the temperature at which it smokes when heated—at that point, any oil is basically ruined. Olive oil generally has a higher smoke point than most other oils, but it is the refined or lower-quality olive oils that have the highest smoke points.

Whether you are using olive oil to sauté, stir-fry, or pan-fry, here are some tips:

- Heat the pan or skillet on medium heat. Once the pan is hot, add the olive oil and heat to just below its smoke point before adding food. The food should sizzle when it's added; if it doesn't, the pan and the oil aren't hot enough.

- Pat food dry before placing it in the oil. This will ensure a crispy exterior.

- Try brushing your meat, seafood, or vegetables with a bit of olive oil when you're grilling or broiling. This will enhance the flavor, seal in the juices, and give you a crispier exterior. And don't forget to brush the grill to keep the food from sticking.

- Use the lower-quality olive oils for stir-frying or pan-frying because they are better for high-heat cooking methods.

- Use olive oil for cooking with foods that contain a high acid content such as vinegar, wine, lemon juice, or tomato to help balance the acidity.

- Add one tablespoon of olive oil to boiling water before adding pasta. This will help to eliminate sticking and clumping.

- Remember that olive oil, although healthy, is also a fat that contains a lot of calories, so use it in moderation.

A Baker's Delight

Most people are used to baking with butter or margarine, but few of us think about olive oil when it comes to baking. Baking with olive oil will give your baked goods a healthier kick, and it can help you to produce lighter-tasting breads, cakes, and other baked goods. Substituting olive oil for butter will drastically reduce the amount of saturated fat and cholesterol in your baked goods. You will also use less fat when baking with olive oil, and that means fewer calories. The best choice for baking is the lite, light, or mild varieties of olive oil because they can stand high heat and have a much milder flavor.

When you are baking or just cooking in general, replacing your bad fats with good ones is easy. When a recipe calls for a vegetable oil or another type of fat like butter or margarine, simply use olive oil instead. As a general guide, substitute an equal amount of olive oil for the same amount of another cooking oil and three-quarters the amount of olive oil when substituting for butter or margarine.

The following substitutions will help you replace butter or margarine with olive oil in your favorite recipes:

Butter/Olive Oil Substitution Chart

Butter	Olive Oil
1 tsp.	¾ tsp.
2 tsp.	1½ tsp.
1 TB.	2¼ tsp.
2 TB.	1½ TB.
¼ cup	3 TB.
⅓ cup	¼ cup
½ cup	¼ cup + 2 TB.
⅔ cup	½ cup
¾ cup	½ cup + 1 TB.
1 cup	¾ cup

The Least You Need to Know

- Olive oil is made from the olive, which is actually a fruit.
- Olive oil is the backbone of the Mediterranean diet.
- Olive oil's primary fat component is monounsaturated fat, which is known for its health benefits. It is low in saturated fats.
- Olive oil contains not only fat but also essential vitamins and antioxidants.
- There are several classifications of olive oil, which are determined by processing method. Some are higher quality than others.
- Olive oil is great for cooking and can even be used in baking.

Wild About Whole Grains

In This Chapter

- The "whole" story
- The foundation of the Mediterranean diet
- What can whole grains do for you?
- Making smart choices
- Whole grains that are traditional to the Mediterranean diet
- Making whole grains a part of your daily diet

Many grain foods are known as comfort foods. Those wonderful complex carbohydrates such as bread, rice, cereal, and pasta make us feel calmed and contented. Throw in the word *whole* and these grain foods are much more than comfort; they are an essential part of a healthy diet. Health experts continually advise that everyone, both young and old, should eat more whole grains. But if whole grains are so healthy, why is it that people eat so few of them? Many people have a good excuse—they don't know exactly what whole grains are and why we should eat them.

What Is a Whole Grain?

All grains are good sources of complex carbohydrates, vitamins, and minerals. However, *whole grains* kick it up a notch by also including more fiber and additional essential nutrients. Whole grains are termed *whole* because they are made up of the entire seed of the grain: the bran, germ, and endosperm. Whole grains can be eaten whole, cracked, split, or ground.

Whole Grains vs. Refined Grains

Grains are broken down into two subgroups: whole grains and refined grains. Whole grains are much better than refined grains for increasing your fiber intake, providing essential nutrients, and contributing to good health.

We already know that a whole-grain food is made from the entire grain kernel. The bran is the outer layer of the grain and supplies antioxidants, B vitamins, trace minerals, and fiber. The germ, nestled inside the endosperm, is tiny but packs a powerful punch, supplying B vitamins, vitamin E, trace minerals, antioxidants, essential fats, and fiber. The endosperm, or the inner part of the grain kernel, contains most of the protein and starchy carbohydrates. The endosperm supplies only small amounts of vitamins and minerals and no fiber.

While whole grains contain all three parts of the kernel, refined grains contain only the endosperm. This is why whole grains contain all the fiber and most of the nutrients. Refined grains are basically whole grains that have been processed or milled and have had the bran and germ removed. Milling provides the grain with a finer texture and improves the shelf life; however, it also strips away dietary fiber, iron, and essential vitamins.

GOOD TO KNOW

When the bran and germ are stripped away, about 25 percent of a grain's protein and most of the key nutrients are lost.

Examples of whole grains include:

- Amaranth
- Barley
- Buckwheat
- Bulgur

- Corn
- Oats, including oatmeal
- Popcorn
- Quinoa

- Rice, wild and brown
- Rye, whole
- Sorghum
- Teff
- Whole-wheat bread, buns, tortillas, crackers, and rolls
- Whole-wheat flour
- Whole-wheat pasta
- Spelt

Examples of refined grains include:

- Baked goods (unless made with a whole-grain flour)
- Crackers made from white or refined flour
- Flour tortillas made from white or refined flour
- White bread, buns, rolls
- White flour
- White pasta or noodles
- White rice

Adding Nutrients Back

Because so many nutrients are stripped away during the milling process of refining grains, most of these grains are enriched, meaning that some of the nutrients that were lost during processing are added back into the food. These are nutrients that were naturally present in the food to begin with. Some B vitamins and iron are added back in, but fiber is not added to enriched grains. This sums up why it is best to choose whole-grain food rather than choosing ones made from refined grains. Shoot for a goal of getting at least half, if not all, of your grains for the day from whole grains.

Whole Grains and the Mediterranean Diet

Whole grains form the foundation of the Mediterranean diet and are included in the largest food section, the plant group, of the Mediterranean Diet Pyramid (see Chapter 3). The pyramid suggests basing every meal on these highly nutritious complex carbohydrates. The more whole grains you include in your daily diet, the more closely you will be following the Mediterranean diet and the more health benefits you will reap.

According to the Whole Grains Council, the average American eats less than one serving of whole grains per day, and 40 percent of Americans eat absolutely no whole grains per day. However, if following the Mediterranean diet is your goal, it's time to set some goals for the consumption of whole grains. Health experts agree that even small amounts of whole grains can put you on the road to better health.

> **TO YOUR HEALTH**
>
> The current U.S. Dietary Guidelines for Americans recommends that all adults eat at least half of their grains as whole grains. That adds up to at least three to five servings of whole grains daily.

Healthy Benefits

The medical evidence speaks for itself—it confirms that whole grains reduce the risk of heart disease, stroke, cancer, and type 2 diabetes. Whole grains can decrease cholesterol, lower your risk for obesity, and help maintain your weight. They have also been associated with a lower incidence of gastrointestinal issues such as constipation and diverticulosis. Studies show that just three servings of whole grains a day can greatly reduce your risk for many chronic diseases. Other health benefits of whole grains include reduced risk for asthma, inflammatory diseases, colon cancer, and hypertension (high blood pressure).

Nutritional Properties of Grains

Whole grains are an abundant source of healthy nutrients. They contain antioxidants (vitamin E and selenium), B vitamins (thiamin, riboflavin, niacin, and folate), and minerals (iron, magnesium, and selenium). In addition, they are packed with dietary fiber and phytonutrients that have antioxidant properties. When all of these nutritional components work together in a whole food, the result is powerful protection for our health.

Choosing Whole Grains

How do you ensure that the foods you are choosing are indeed whole grain? Whole grains currently take up about 10 to 15 percent of grocery shelves. It can sometimes be a challenge for consumers to find these healthier whole grains amongst the sea of refined-grain foods.

The key is to check labels carefully. Don't be fooled by the color of a product or certain wording. For example, just because a loaf of bread is brown in color does not necessarily mean it is made from whole-wheat flour and is, therefore, a whole grain.

Many times breads labeled wheat are actually colored with molasses or caramel coloring, or they are made with a mixture of both refined and whole-wheat flours, where proportions vary. You may come across the words *multi-grain*, *stone-ground*, *cracked wheat*, *100 percent wheat* (meaning wheat is used, but not necessarily whole wheat), *bran*, or *seven grain*, just to name a few. These might sound nutritious, but unfortunately, they do not guarantee a whole-grain product—and often they are not whole grain.

To determine if a food product actually is whole grain and contains whole-grain ingredients, look for the word *whole* on the package, such as *whole wheat* or *whole grain*, and check to see if whole grains appear among the first items in the ingredient list. Not all whole grains have the word *whole*, so look for other whole-grain ingredients such as brown rice, bulgur, graham flour, oatmeal, and wild rice.

Use the Nutrition Facts Panel (see Chapter 5) to choose foods with a higher Percent Daily Value (%DV) for fiber. The more fiber a food has, the better chance there is that a good amount of whole grains can be found in the product. If the product has 20 percent or more %DV for fiber, it's considered a high-fiber food. You can also check for a whole-grain authorized health claim by the FDA on the label that states, "Diets rich in whole-grain foods and other plant foods that are low in total fat, saturated fat, and cholesterol may reduce the risk of heart disease and certain cancers." Foods that display this specific claim must contain at least 51 percent or more whole grains by weight and be low in fat.

HEALTHY MORSELS

The Whole Grains Council has developed two Whole Grain Stamps to help consumers easily find whole-grain foods. You can currently find the stamps on hundreds of foods with more to come. Food products that bear the Whole Grain Stamp must contain at least 8 grams of whole grains per serving, which equals half a serving of whole grains. Products that bear the 100% Whole Grain Stamp must contain at least 16 grams of whole grains per serving, which equals a full serving of whole grains.

Discovering the Grains of the Mediterranean

There are lots of whole grains out there for you to try, and many are traditional to the Mediterranean diet. Now is the time to tantalize your taste buds and begin sampling some of these tasty whole grains. There are many grains you might already be familiar with such as rice, cereal, pasta, and breads, but there are many more that may be new to you. A little information on these whole grains may make them less scary and a lot more manageable!

Whole-Wheat Bulgur

Bulgur is a whole grain with a mild, nutty flavor and is a staple in the Mediterranean diet. It is cracked wheat that has been partially cooked to be quick cooking. Bulgur is especially high in fiber, protein, and minerals, but is low in calories and fat. In fact, bulgur contains more fiber than oats, buckwheat, or corn. This versatile grain comes in three grinds: fine, medium, and coarse. The finest grind of bulgur is perfect for hot breakfast cereals and desserts. The medium-size grind is preferred for grain salads such as tabbouleh salad, stews, soups, and multi-grain baked goods. The coarsely ground bulgur can be used for pilaf, stuffing, and casseroles. Bulgur makes a great meat extender and, because of its high protein content, a nutritious meat substitute in meatless meals. Bulgur is used much like rice in the Mediterranean diet and combines well with many other foods.

Hulled Barley

Barley is a cereal grain that is only lightly milled and retains much of its soluble and insoluble fiber. With hulled barley, only the outermost hull of the grain is removed, which makes for a chewier grain and a more nutritious whole-grain food. In fact, hulled barley is the only form of barley that is considered a whole grain. Varieties such as scotch barley and barley oats retain more of the bran than pearled barley, but none of these forms are considered a whole grain. Hulled barley makes a healthy choice for use in grain salads, soups, risotto, and stews, or as a stuffing for vegetables. It has a wonderful chewy texture, making an interesting addition to your meals. It can be a nice alternative to rice.

Whole-Grain Couscous

Whole-grain couscous is a coarsely ground semolina pasta made from whole-grain durum flour. It is not always made from whole grains, so be sure it is labeled as either whole wheat or whole grain. It's widely used in Middle Eastern countries but is becoming much more popular in American dishes. Couscous has a light flavor and is very similar to rice in shape, color, and texture. In fact, it is almost a perfect mixture of both rice and pasta. Couscous absorbs the flavors of Mediterranean foods such as herbs, spices, vegetables, stews, lamb, seafood, or chicken very nicely.

Polenta

Polenta is a common food in the Mediterranean region and is a must when discussing whole grains. Polenta is made from ground cornmeal; however, you want to avoid de-germinated cornmeal as this has the germ removed and is therefore not a whole grain. Your best bet is to buy stone-ground, whole-grain cornmeal and use that to make polenta to ensure you have a whole-grain product. The word *polenta* can be used to refer to the dish or to the actual ground cornmeal itself. To make polenta, cornmeal is boiled in water to make a porridge-type dish—something that is better known in America as cornmeal mush. Traditionally polenta can take some time to prepare; however, a form of quick-cooking polenta is gaining popularity. After polenta is cooked, it can be left in the refrigerator overnight to allow it to harden into a doughlike texture. At that point, it can be baked and cut into squares almost like cornbread. Polenta can be served in numerous ways: baked, in stews, and as a bread substitute. Cooked polenta can be used much like pasta as a base for sauces, toppings, vegetables, seafood, and meats.

Quinoa

Quinoa may not be well known in most American kitchens, but it is quite popular with the people of the Mediterranean. Quinoa is light and fluffy, with a slightly crunchy texture and nutty flavor when cooked. It is quite high in protein and antioxidants compared to other whole grains. In fact, it has nearly twice the amount of protein as other grains and it's considered a *complete protein*, making it a great choice as a meat substitute or for use in vegetarian diets. This grain is a high-fiber food with a whopping five grams of fiber per cooked cup. Quinoa is very versatile and can be eaten as a breakfast cereal, mixed with vegetables, or added to soups, stews, and salads. It can also be used to make flour for breads or used as a substitution for pasta, couscous, or rice.

> **DEFINITION**
>
> A **complete protein** (or whole protein) provides the body with an adequate proportion of all nine essential amino acids needed for optimal health. Most complete proteins come from animal sources such as meats, seafood, and dairy products, with very few coming from plant sources.

Flours to Discover

Most of us think about white all-purpose flour for baking and that is what probably sits on most of our pantry shelves. White all-purpose flour is made from wheat that has been refined, stripping away the layers that contain all the nutrients, and therefore is not a whole grain. In other words, it is wheat flour, but not whole-wheat flour—and as we've discussed, the nutritional difference between refined and whole-grain flours is quite significant.

Refined flours are not the type of flour that you would find in most homes around the Mediterranean. Many different whole-grain flours have a much higher nutritional content and create a more complex taste and heartier texture because they include the bran and germ of the grain. The good news is that these flours can work just fine in your favorite dishes and baked goods.

Whole-grain flours don't last as long as refined flour, so when buying them, be sure to check the sell-by date to buy the freshest available. They should be stored in the refrigerator or freezer in an airtight container (be sure to set flour out and get it to room temperature before using it). You can expect most of them to last about three months so only buy what you will use in that time. Whole-grain flours can cook differently than white all-purpose flour, so you may have to alter recipes slightly to get the end product you are looking for.

Here are some tips to help you add whole-grain goodness to your cooking and baking:

- Use whole-grain flour in simple recipes that you have made before and in recipes that call for only a small amount of flour. It might be helpful at first to find recipes that actually call for whole-grain flour.

- Research online or in cookbooks which flours work best for different foods or baked goods (such as breads versus cakes). You can get started with the list of flours later in this chapter.

- Start slow by substituting at least half of all-purpose flour with whole-grain flours such as spelt or whole-wheat flour.

- Because whole-wheat flours absorb more liquid than refined white flour, you may need to add additional liquid in small portions, a little at a time, to get the consistency you need.

- Sift flour before and after measuring to help improve texture.

- You may need to use more leavening agent (such as baking powder or baking soda) to help with the rising properties of whole-grain flour.

- Put a pan of water in the oven while baking to help retain moisture; whole-grain flour tends to be drier than other kinds of flour.

- Because many whole-grain flours are *gluten*-free, if you are baking bread leavened with yeast, you need half of the flour you use to be a gluten-containing flour.

DEFINITION

Gluten is a starch that is found in wheat. It's what gives breads the elasticity and structure that allow it to rise. High-gluten flours are best used for breads. Baked goods that use baking powder or baking soda as leaveners such as muffins, quick breads, and cakes do not need gluten to rise. Flours with less gluten work well in these types of baked goods.

With a little practice you will be able to find the combinations of refined flours and whole-grain flours that suit your needs. By adding some whole-grain flour to white all-purpose flour, you can begin to add fiber and other essential nutrients to your favorite baked goods. The more you know about the different whole-grain flours, the easier it will be to work with them.

Whole-Wheat Flour

Whole-wheat flour has a high gluten content and a coarse texture. It is sometimes referred to as whole-wheat bread flour and is ideal for bread baking due to its ability to rise. Whole-wheat flour is higher in fiber and protein than refined white flour. Because bread made with 100 percent whole-wheat flour can be somewhat coarse and heavy and doesn't keep long, it's best to mix in refined flour (30 to 50 percent) to lighten the texture. Your bread will taste better and you will still be getting the benefit of using a whole grain.

Spelt Flour

Spelt flour is close in flavor and texture to whole-wheat flour. It contains no wheat but does contain some gluten. However, the gluten in spelt is a bit fragile so it's important not to overmix your dough or batter since gluten provides elasticity and structure to baked goods. Spelt is a popular and easy substitute for wheat flour in most breads, baked goods, and other recipes. It is a bit nuttier and sweeter than whole-wheat flour, is high in protein, and has a strong nutritional profile.

Barley Flour

Barley flour is a delicate, low-gluten flour that is made by grinding whole barley. This flour is moist and has a sweet, nutlike flavor. As with many other whole-grain flours, it can be used to replace part of the wheat flour (white or refined flour) in baked goods and recipes to provide a unique flavor and texture as well as a kick of nutrition. Try substituting $\frac{1}{3}$ cup of barley flour in place of your regular flour for a more tender product. Barley flour can also serve as a thickener in soups and sauces.

Whole Rye Flour

Rye flour is milled from whole rye berries and grains of rye grass. It provides moisture and density to baked goods and is low in gluten content. Rye flour can be bought in a variety of colors: dark, medium, and light. The color will depend on how much bran is removed during the milling process. Dark rye flour, the least-refined form of rye flour, is high in nutrients—even higher than whole-wheat flour. Pumpernickel flour is a type of dark rye flour that is used to make pumpernickel bread. The medium-colored rye flour is most common and is still quite nutritious, because most of the bran is left. Equal proportions of rye and wheat flour (white or refined flour) work well in yeasted and quick breads to help the rising process. Rye flour has a slightly sour taste, making it a great flour to use for rye bread and sourdough bread. Light rye flour is the most refined or has the most bran removed, making it the least nutritious.

Cooking Whole Grains

You can add whole grains daily without cooking simply by choosing whole-grain breads, cereals, and other prepared whole-grain foods. However, that isn't the only way to include and enjoy them. You can include them in many of your favorite dishes and recipes by making easy substitutions. Because some of these whole grains may be a little different than what you're used to, here are some guidelines:

- Cooking most whole grains is very similar to the process for cooking rice. Put the dry grain in a pan of water or broth, bring to a boil, and then simmer until the liquid is absorbed. Cooking times will vary depending on the grain type, so read package directions.

- For grains that are tougher and take longer to cook, let them presoak in the allotted amount of water for a few hours before cooking.

- Try batch cooking when you cook grains. They will keep at least three to four days in the refrigerator, and they take just a few minutes to warm up. You can toss them into salads, stews, and soups.

- Look for quick-cooking grains now on the market, such as instant brown rice—but make sure you are buying a whole-grain product. Review the Nutrition Facts Panel to ensure you are getting the fiber you expect.

Tips for Going Whole Grain

If you want to follow the Mediterranean diet, then it's time to start adding those healthy whole grains to your daily diet. Be adventurous and try some whole grains that you've never tasted and maybe have never heard of. Forget the myths that whole grains don't taste good or that they are difficult to work into your daily diet. You'll be pleasantly surprised at how wrong these myths are—but you won't know until you try!

Here are some tips to get you started:

- Try rolled oats, barley, buckwheat, or other whole grains as your breakfast cereal topped with fresh fruit.

- Substitute a mixture of unrefined whole-grain flour for refined flour in your baked goods and as thickeners.

- Step up your breakfast foods by making pancakes or muffins using a combination of whole-grain flours.

- Don't restrict yourself to the same whole grains every day. As with other food groups, variety is best. This will ensure you are receiving the most nutritional benefits from all types of whole grains.

- Choose whole-grain breads and cereals. Making simple changes like whole-grain breakfast cereal instead of a refined, sugary cereal and whole-wheat bread in place of white bread can make big changes to your nutritional intake.

- Try whole-grain rice and other side dishes. This is a simple change and can really add flavor to your dishes. You might be surprised at how much better brown rice tastes than white rice, for example. Add something new to your pilaf or other side dishes like couscous, barley, or bulgur.

- Try buying whole-grain pasta or a pasta that is a blend of whole-grain and white flours. Use them with your favorite sauces or in casseroles, soups, and cold salads.

- Check out new recipes from sources like the Whole Grains Council (wholegrainscouncil.com/) to sharpen your whole-grain cooking skills.

- Short on time? Add cooked bulgur, brown or wild rice, whole-wheat couscous, or barley to your favorite canned or homemade soup—an instant serving of whole grains!

- Jazz up your bread stuffing with cooked bulgur, wild rice, or barley.

- Add ¾ cup of uncooked oats to each pound of ground turkey or ground chicken breast to make meatballs, stuffed peppers, burgers, or meatloaf. Whole grains add flavor and make a great meat extender.

- Stir in a handful of oats to your plain, nonfat yogurt along with some fruit.

- Do something simple like snacking on popcorn. What could be easier than air-popped popcorn? Just be sure it isn't covered in fat and salt.

- Use oat bran as a coating for fish or chicken.

The key is to begin finding ways to fit those whole grains in anywhere you can. It doesn't take a lot of whole grains to get what is recommended daily, but shoot for as many as you can. Always check food labels and ingredients lists to ensure you are actually buying a whole-grain product. Continue learning about and trying a variety of whole grains.

The Least You Need to Know

- The foundation of the Mediterranean diet is built on plant foods, including whole grains.
- A whole grain by definition includes the whole seeds: bran, germ, and endosperm.
- Whole grains are much more nutritious than refined grains and are packed with fiber.
- Foods need to include the word *whole,* in most cases, if they are actually a whole grain. Always read food labels and the ingredient list.
- Don't be afraid to cook and bake with whole grains, and try to find new ways to add them to your daily diet. They can be tasty and nutritious and add some wonderful new flavors.

Fabulous Fruits

In This Chapter

- Fruit's place in the Mediterranean diet
- The nutritional beauty of fruit
- The fruitful way to improve your health
- Fruits of the Mediterranean and beyond
- Fresh, frozen, canned, or dried
- Increasing your fruit intake

Fruit is one of the most natural foods in the world and is one that most of us take for granted. It is abundant in variety, is readily available, and provides a sweet goodness. However, studies show that 90 percent of Americans don't eat enough fruit. Eating a colorful variety of fruits can provide a wide range of valuable nutrients that are essential for good health. There are proven links that eating more fruit can lead to lowered risk for some chronic conditions. No wonder fruit is a major component of the Mediterranean diet.

Fruit and the Mediterranean Diet

You might be starting to notice a pattern: every time we discuss a plant-based food, we mention the foundation of the Mediterranean Diet Pyramid (see Chapter 3), because plant-based foods are what this diet is based on. The recommendation is to base every meal on these healthy plant foods, and that includes fruit. The key is to include fruit as often as possible and to consume a wide variety to ensure you get the most of their nutritional benefits. You might be surprised to learn that some of the fruits included in this group within the Mediterranean Diet Pyramid include olives, avocados, dates, and pomegranates. However, there are also many more familiar fruits such as strawberries, apples, grapes, and pears.

> **TO YOUR HEALTH**
>
> Fruit is a healthy and natural source of energy. Forget that midday candy bar or cup of coffee as a pick-me-up—grab a piece of fresh fruit instead. It's loaded with good nutrition instead of empty calories.

Healthy Benefits

No matter what the fruit, whether it's native to the Mediterranean region or is more common on American grocery shelves, they are simply a healthy food. Eating more fruit as part of an overall healthy diet has been shown to reduce the risk of stroke, cardiovascular diseases, type 2 diabetes, and certain cancers such as colon and stomach cancers. In addition, digestive problems such as constipation and diarrhea can possibly be alleviated by eating more fruit. With the natural fiber that fruit contains, it can help to regulate bowel movements. When you make the simple change of eating fruit in place of sweets, junk foods, or other foods with added sugar and fat, you may even lose weight or better maintain a healthy weight.

Nutritional Properties of Fruit

Mother Nature placed plenty of health secrets inside fruit. Fruit is naturally low in fat, sodium, and calories and as a bonus contains absolutely no cholesterol, saturated fat, or trans fats. Most fruit contains about 80 percent water, so fruit even contributes to your overall daily fluid intake. Most fruit is rich in potassium, which is helpful in maintaining a healthy blood pressure. Some of the most valuable nutrients found in fruit include dietary fiber and antioxidants such as vitamin C and vitamin A. Eating a variety of colorful fruits can provide plenty of phytonutrients such as flavonoids, carotenoids, and phenols—all of which can improve your health and lower your risk for various chronic health conditions. Mixing things up and consuming a variety of fruits will incorporate a broader range of nutrient consumption in your diet—so think variety and color!

Ever wonder why fruit tastes so sweet? That would be the work of something called fructose—the natural sugar found in fruit. In this day and age, we are taught to think of sugar as something to avoid or limit; however, there are many different types of sugar. There are naturally occurring sugars, like the fructose in fruit and the lactose in dairy products. Then there are added sugars, like those added to cookies, baked goods, soft drinks, and other processed foods. The difference is that the naturally occurring sugars found in whole natural foods, like fruits and dairy products, are loaded with essential nutrients for good health. On the other hand, added sugars, which are refined sugars, are usually found in foods that provide empty calories and little or no nutritional value. So even though you may hear the word *sugar*, when it comes to eating fruit, you are doing a good thing for your body.

GOOD TO KNOW

In the body, the natural sugar in fruit acts the same way as added sugar. Our bodies don't know the difference, so for some diabetics, this could pose a problem. However, if you are diabetic, it's important to strategically include fruit in your meal plan for managing diabetes. Fruit is high in fiber, which can help to delay the absorption of sugar into the bloodstream and help to maintain blood sugar levels. Speak with a registered dietitian or certified diabetes educator about how to include fruit in your meal plan.

Popular Fruits of the Mediterranean

You already know that fruit is a vital part of the Mediterranean diet. But can you name some of the fruits that are most popular in those regions? Some could be fruits you already enjoy and others might be something new and exciting to try! Let's take a closer look at a few of the more popular ones.

Olives

Olives are the fruit of the olive tree. The olive, as well as olive oil, are staples of the Mediterranean diet (see Chapter 6). In fact, although olives are grown all over the world, the primary source continues to be the Mediterranean region. They are far too bitter to be consumed in their natural state, right off the tree, and require some processing (fermentation or curing) before they are considered edible. The color of olives depends on their ripeness as well as the method of processing used. You can find the unripe green olives or the fully ripened black variety. Olives are small but plentiful in heart-healthy monounsaturated fats, vitamin E, iron, copper, a variety of beneficial phytonutrients, and even some fiber. You can use olives in salads, on pizza, in pasta dishes or main dishes, as a pre-dinner appetizer (as they often do in the Mediterranean), or just by themselves as a snack. Varieties of olives used include Kalamata, Manzanilla, Sicilian, and Gaeta. Keep in mind that they can be high in sodium and are quite high in fat, unlike most other fruits, so they are best eaten in moderation.

Avocados

Many think of avocados as a vegetable because they don't have the same sweet flavor that most fruits do, but they are undoubtedly a fruit—and one that is quite popular in the Mediterranean regions. They pack a powerful nutritional punch compared to other fruits because they have especially high levels of protein, fiber, niacin, thiamin, riboflavin, folate, vitamin E, zinc, potassium, magnesium, and numerous phytonutrients. Avocados are cholesterol- and sodium-free and as a bonus, most of an avocado's calories come from heart-healthy monounsaturated fat. Because of their relatively higher fat content—about 5 grams of fat per serving—they tend to be high in calories, so moderation is the key for this nutrient-dense fruit.

Avocados will ripen after they have been picked, so buy ones that are a bit under-ripe, meaning one that is firm but not rock hard. Give it a quick squeeze and it should give a little; if it is too soft it is overripe. You can store avocados at room temperature in a brown paper bag for about three to four days until they ripen and soften up a bit. Once they are ripened, you can store them in the refrigerator until you eat them for about two to three more days. Avocados can be used in salads, on sandwiches, in creams, in cold soups, and for well-known dishes like guacamole. Do not cook avocados, except maybe to warm them up a bit, as this makes them bitter.

With all of the healthy components of avocados, they may help to lower blood pressure and reduce the risk of high blood pressure, stroke, and heart disease. In addition, avocados are known to be a substantial source of lutein (a type of phytonutrient called a carotenoid), which comes from the yellow pigment in the avocado. Lutein has been shown to help maintain eye health as we age.

TO YOUR HEALTH

To prepare an avocado, start with a washed and ripened avocado and cut it lengthwise all the way around the pit. Rotate or twist the halves to separate. Slide the tip of a spoon underneath the pit and gently lift it out. To remove the peel, place the cut side down and starting at the small end, remove the skin with a butter knife, a spoon, or your fingers.

Figs

Figs come from the ficus tree and are believed to have originated in western Asia, but they eventually found their way to the Mediterranean. The best-quality figs are grown and produced in the Mediterranean regions where it is dry and warm, although California has since gotten in on the action.

Figs come in two forms: fresh and dried. Dried figs are most common because fresh figs do not transport well and, once picked, do not last very long. Dried figs contain abundant amounts of calcium, iron, fiber, protein, and potassium as well as two phytonutrients (flavonoids and polyphenols). They contain absolutely no fat, sodium, or cholesterol. They make a great sweet and nutritious snack and, considering their unique flavor and texture, pair well with meat, poultry, fish, stews, and vegetables. Figs make a flavorful and nutritious contribution to cookies and other baked goods; in fact, figs contain a natural chemical, humectant, which absorbs water and will extend the freshness and moistness in baked products. Fig purée can make the perfect substitute for fat in many baked good recipes. You can store dried figs in unopened packages in the cupboard for up to six months. Once the package is opened, they should be refrigerated and stored in a container with a tight-fitting lid. Fresh figs won't last long at room temperature, so they should be stored in the refrigerator, where they will last for several days.

TO YOUR HEALTH

One small quantity of dried figs, $1/4$ cup, provides 5 grams of fiber, which is 20 percent of the recommended daily value.

Pomegranates

Pomegranates, although hugely popular in the Mediterranean region, are just beginning to become one of the hot new superfoods around the world. This little red fruit is further proof that the Mediterranean diet is one of the healthiest diets around. What is it about this tasty fruit that adds to the health benefits of the Mediterranean diet? Why are they stirring up such a buzz in other areas? Pomegranates, especially the juice, contain several phytonutrients including tannins, polyphenols, and anthocyanins. In fact, pomegranate juice contains more antioxidants and phytonutrients than red wine or green tea. Research has pointed to these antioxidants and phytonutrients as being beneficial in helping to protect the body from several chronic diseases such as heart disease, rheumatoid arthritis, and certain cancers. New research has found that certain phytonutrients in pomegranates may even reduce the risk of a type of breast cancer called hormone-dependent breast cancer. In addition, the nutrients in this fruit can help slow the aging process and neutralize free radicals, which can damage body cells, tissues, and DNA and cause chronic health issues. Pomegranates are low in calories and a good source of fiber, vitamin C, calcium, potassium, and iron.

Pomegranates take a little bit more work than other fruits. After cutting the leathery outer skin and peeling it back, you will find the seeds of the fruit, or arils. You can pick out the arils, with their sweet-tart flavor, and store them in the refrigerator to enjoy in salads, yogurt, sauces, and almost anything else you can think of to add a powerful health punch. You can pick out about $\frac{1}{2}$ to $\frac{3}{4}$ cup of seeds from a medium-size pomegranate. During the winter months when the cold-weather produce starts to become boring, these little red fruits—which only make an appearance as fresh fruit September through January—can really spice up your fruit life. Whether you use the seeds or drink the juice of the pomegranate, you are doing your body a healthy favor.

GOOD TO KNOW

If you take medication on a regular basis, talk to your doctor before trying these tasty fruits; pomegranate juice can interfere with the metabolism of many medications.

Dates

Another popular fruit in the Mediterranean is dates. This fruit is available in stores year-round and can be purchased soft, semi-dried, and dried. In the Mediterranean, desserts and snacks rely heavily on dried fruits such as dates because of their intensely sweet flavor. This fruit is virtually fat-free as well as cholesterol- and sodium-free. They contain few calories yet are rich in fiber and boast a vast amount of nutrients essential for optimal health including vitamin C, vitamin K, vitamin A, calcium, iron, potassium, manganese, magnesium, and copper. They are rich in the B-complex vitamins, containing B_6, niacin, pantothenic acid, and riboflavin. In addition, this sweet fruit contains many of the health-promoting phytonutrients such as tannins, beta-carotene, lutein, and zeaxanthin. The phytonutrients found in this fruit help protect the body from free radicals and can help protect against certain cancers. In addition, dates have some anti-infective, anti-inflammatory, and anti-hemorrhagic properties. Dates are even said to be an excellent treatment for intestinal problems and also have a laxative effect.

Look for fresh dates in the produce section of the supermarket, or find dried dates near the raisins and prunes. Fresh dates should be stored in a well-sealed container. They can last up to two months at room temperature or up to eight months in the refrigerator. Store them in the freezer and they will last for several years. Dried dates will last up to a year if refrigerated. Whether you are choosing fresh or dried dates look for plump fruit with a skin that is unbroken and appears smoothly wrinkled. If your dates have been stored for a while and look dried out, put them in a bowl of warm water for several minutes.

Just a small amount of chopped dates can bring a ton of flavor to so many dishes such as salads, dressings, sauces, gravies, toppings, syrups, and more. Dried or soft dates can be eaten plain for a sweet snack. They can also be stuffed with almonds, walnuts, or cream cheese.

Everyday Alternatives

While some of the fancier, more exotic fruits of the Mediterranean are undoubtedly nutritious, new, and exciting, don't overlook the everyday fruits that are native to your area. They, too, can be nutritional powerhouses and are tops for great value, availability, and flavor. In fact, many of these fruits are indeed the same fruits that are eaten on a daily basis in the Mediterranean.

Strawberries

After a long winter of dutifully fulfilling your fruit intake with the limited number of fruits available, strawberries and other berries can be a long-awaited delight for your taste buds. Strawberries are just as common to the Mediterranean as they are in the United States. This fruit has a lot more to offer than just their sweet, delicious flavor. They are low in calories and high in fiber, especially soluble fiber. They include essential nutrients such as folate, vitamin C, manganese, and potassium, just to name a few. You may be surprised to learn that a serving of about eight medium strawberries contains more vitamin C than an orange. The anthocyanins in strawberries are the phytonutrients that provides its rich, red color and have been shown to serve as a potent antioxidant that helps to protect cell structures in the body and prevent oxidative damage in the body's organ system. Strawberries are also quite high in a phytonutrient known as phenols, making them a heart-protective fruit, an anti-cancer fruit, and an anti-inflammatory fruit all rolled into one.

To get the full nutritional benefit, it is best to enjoy strawberries when they are in season from April to July. In addition, purchasing them from local markets will ensure an even higher nutritional value, because fruits begin to lose nutrients soon after they are picked. Strawberries are highly perishable and should be purchased only a few days prior to use. It is best to store strawberries in a colander in the refrigerator to let air circulate around them. You can also find special containers on the market that allow air to circulate around fruit when stored; these are great for storing strawberries. Remove the caps from strawberries only after you wash them and right before eating them.

> **TO YOUR HEALTH**
>
> Don't forget other berries such as blueberries, raspberries, and blackberries—all of which are high on the nutritional score sheet.

Grapes

Grapes are common in both the Mediterranean diet and the typical Western diet. American varieties are available mostly in the months of September and October while the European varieties are available all year long. Grapes are full of beneficial nutrients such as manganese, potassium, vitamin C, thiamin, and B_6, but studies show that red grapes get their health benefits from a category of phytonutrients called polyphenols. The three types of polyphenols in grapes (found mostly in the skins and seeds of the fruit) with the biggest health benefits are flavonoids, phenolic acids, and resveratrol. Flavonoids are what provide grapes, grape juice, and red wines with their vibrant purple color. The darker the grapes are, the higher their concentration of flavonoids. Flavonoids, phenolic acids, and resveratrol all help to decrease the risk of heart disease and stroke. Red grapes also contain anthocyanins, tannins, carotenes, inositol, and other health protective phytonutrients.

Grapes are simple fruits and, best of all, require no more prep time than a simple washing. They make a great snack or addition to salads. For a cool treat in the hot months, try freezing and eating your grapes. Because grapes are quite perishable, always store them in the refrigerator.

Oranges

Oranges are part of the citrus fruit family. They are a winter fruit (October to February) and contain high levels of vitamin C, potassium, vitamin A, and B-complex vitamins. Peel into one juicy orange and you can fulfill your daily requirement for vitamin C. Oranges are bursting with healthy doses of beneficial antioxidants and phytonutrients such as beta-carotene, flavonoids, and lutein, which appear to help reduce inflammation, lower cholesterol and blood pressure, and reduce the risk for heart disease. They are high in soluble fiber and low in calories—but only if you stick to the whole fruit instead of juice. Once oranges are juiced, much of the pulp, and therefore the fiber, is gone. In addition, many store-bought juices contain added sugar, preservatives, and other artificial ingredients.

Oranges can be kept at room temperature, but they keep better and longer—up to two weeks—in the refrigerator. Oranges make a satisfying sweet snack and are a great addition to a green salad. Try mixing chopped oranges with plain, low-fat vanilla yogurt and a sprinkle of almonds or walnuts for the perfect Mediterranean-style snack.

Apples

Apples come in many varieties, and all are low in calories, contain no fat or sodium, and are big on flavor. You can find just about any flavor to fit your taste buds—from tart to sweet and everything in between. We have all been told that "An apple a day keeps the doctor away," but the question is, "Why?" It's partly due to its long list of phytonutrients that function as antioxidants as well as flavonoids and phenolic acids that support heart health. Apples are also full of vitamin C. Several studies have associated eating apples with a reduced risk of some types of cancers, heart disease, asthma, and type 2 diabetes.

One of the apple's strongest nutritional attributes is its fiber content. Just a small apple can provide about 3 to 5 grams of fiber. However, keep in mind that the fiber, as well as many of the antioxidants and phytonutrients, is located in the fruit's skin, so peeling the apple will remove most of the health benefits. Whole apples are a much better nutritional choice than apple juice, because the juice lacks fiber and other phytonutrients and may contain some added sugars. Apples should be quite firm when you purchase them and should be stored in the refrigerator for better retention of nutrients.

Apples are another simple fruit that take nothing but a washing to prepare. However, in addition to eating them raw, you can add them to salads, baked goods, or stuffing. Apples make a delicious duo with protein foods such as cheese, peanut butter, or chicken.

Fruit: The New Dessert

Fruit is truly nature's candy—naturally sweet and filled with every imaginable nutrient needed for good health. In the Mediterranean, fresh fruit is the typical, and preferred, daily dessert. People of the Mediterranean regions rarely consume high-calorie, high-sugar, and fat-laden desserts. Fresh fruit can help to satisfy that momentary craving for something sweet after a meal, and it is good for your health.

Other than simply grabbing a fresh piece of fruit, there are many other ways to enjoy fruit as a dessert. With all of the varieties of fruits available, you would be hard-pressed to not find some wonderful fruity desserts. Grilled fruit is just one example and is a delicious treat for a summertime meal. Check out the wonderful fruit dessert recipes in Chapter 22 for more ideas.

HEALTHY MORSELS

Many people are under the impression that fruit is too expensive to enjoy daily. That is far from the truth when you compare how much money you spend on other foods, especially junk foods. Replace those foods with fruit and you won't be spending any extra bucks. In fact, you might even save money by buying fruits that are in season at your local market. However, you should buy only what you will eat within a few days so that you are not wasting fruit and throwing money away.

Fresh Isn't the Only Option

There are numerous ways you can enjoy fruit—fresh is only one option. You can get the fruit you need in other forms, including frozen, canned, and dried. In fact, the nutrients in some fresh fruit can begin to deteriorate as soon as they are picked. If you're not buying local, and the fruit has been sitting a long time in the store, much of the nutritional value may have been lost. However, most frozen and canned fruit (as well as vegetables) are processed within hours of harvest so that much of their flavor and nutritional value are preserved. This doesn't mean that frozen and canned are always best, but they are an option when your favorite fresh fruit is out of season or you don't have it in the house. Stocking your kitchen with all types of fruit will ensure you always have some on hand. The one problem with canned and frozen fruit is that they may include added sugar, so be sure to check food labels. Buy canned fruits that are canned in water or their own juices rather than syrup, and look for frozen fruits that are unsweetened.

The other option, and it is a good one, is dried fruits. There is a wide variety of dried fruits including raisins, apples, apricots, bananas, cherries, cranberries, dates, figs, pineapples, and plums (prunes), to name a few. Compared to their fresh counterparts, dried fruits have a much longer shelf life and usually contain more fiber, iron, potassium, and selenium. However, with that comes a higher calorie and carbohydrate content in the form of natural sugar, so serving sizes are much smaller. Dried fruits tend to lose some vitamins, such as B vitamins and vitamin C, as they are destroyed when the fruit is dried. Some manufacturers will add these vitamins back; check for this information on the food's nutrition label. Sulfur is also something that is often added to dried fruits to preserve color. You will find *Contains Sulfites* on the label for those people who are sulfite-sensitive. Dried fruit makes a great snack, or you can use it to top hot or cold cereals and yogurt. You can add them to baked goods, stuffing, salads, trail mix, and couscous or other grains. Be aware that some dried fruit may have added sugar. For example, sugar is often added to dried cranberries because they are so tart; few people would eat them if they didn't have added sugar. It may add a few more calories, but it doesn't take away from the nutritional content of dried fruit. The bottom line is that canned, frozen, and dried fruits are there to complement, not replace, your daily intake of fruits—they are simply another option. Choose fresh when possible, but keep other forms in mind.

TO YOUR HEALTH

Fruit juices can be another option for fruit intake; however, they are not normally recommended because the majority of fiber and other nutrients are removed in processing. If using fruit juices, use them only occasionally and make sure the label states 100 percent juice with no added sugars. Of course, there will be naturally occurring sugars in the product. If you are using grape juice as an alternative to wine, drink it in moderation and ensure it is 100 percent juice with no added sugar.

Tips for Including More Fruit

Experts suggest that you consume at least five to nine total servings of fruits and vegetables every day. By adding plenty of fruit to your daily diet, you will be tapping into a rich source of nutrients that will help to protect your health. The good news is that it might not be as hard as you think to consume all the fruit that you need. Here are some tips to help you get more fruit into your daily routine.

- Make fruit convenient by keeping some washed and ready to be eaten in the refrigerator. The easier it is, the better chance it will be eaten.

- Use fresh or dried fruit for quick snacks, especially when you have a sweet tooth. Fruit travels well and makes the perfect on-the-go snack.

- Sneak fruit into meals. Add dried cranberries to green salads, peaches or pineapple to your baked ham, blueberries to your favorite pancake recipe, or chopped dates to muffins. The ideas are endless.

- Start your day with fruit by adding it to your hot or cold breakfast cereal, eating it plain, or mixing it into a smoothie.

- Add fresh or dried fruit to plain yogurt.

- Add fresh or dried fruit to your green salads for a well-balanced, satisfying lunch or dinner. With so many combinations of fruits and vegetables, you can make a completely different salad for every day of the week.

- Do as they do in the Mediterranean and serve fruit-based desserts.

- Widen your horizon and wake up your taste buds with new fruits.

The Least You Need to Know

- Fruit is a plant-based food and one of the foundations of the Mediterranean Diet Pyramid.

- Eating plenty of fruit as part of an overall healthy diet can help lower your risk for stroke, heart disease, type 2 diabetes, and certain cancers. It can also help you to meet your daily fluid intake.

- Fruits are full of vitamins, minerals, fiber, antioxidants, and phytonutrients, all of which are important for good health.

- Popular fruits of the Mediterranean include olives, avocados, figs, pomegranates, and dates. However, you don't need to get fancy as long as you are eating a variety of fruit each day.

- Dried, canned, and frozen fruits are additional options if fresh fruit isn't available, but try to use fresh as often as possible.

Vital Vegetables

In This Chapter

- How veggies fit into the Mediterranean diet
- Boost your health with vegetables
- All that veggies have to offer
- A closer look at a few common Mediterranean veggies
- Beyond iceberg: the super greens
- Time to increase your veggie intake

I bet your mom always told you to eat your vegetables! She might not have known exactly why you needed to eat them every day, but she had the right idea. This chapter clues you in to why vegetables need to be part of your everyday life and why they are such a significant component of the Mediterranean diet. You would be hard-pressed to declare you don't like vegetables when they come in such a variety of colors, flavors, and textures. Vegetables offer valuable nutrients that are absolutely essential for good health. Years of research prove that eating more vegetables can lead to lowering the risk for some chronic health conditions.

Connection to the Mediterranean Diet

The foundation of the Mediterranean diet is the plant-based group, and it includes vegetables in a big way. The recommendation of the Mediterranean Diet Pyramid (see Chapter 3) is to base every meal on healthy plant foods, including vegetables. That means doing your best to eat them at every meal and even as snacks when possible. The key, as with fruits, is to eat a large variety and a rainbow of colors to get the mix of nutrients your body needs.

Mediterranean cuisine incorporates loads of vegetables. There are many typical vegetables from the Mediterranean regions that may seem more unusual to you; however, it isn't only these vegetables that will provide health benefits. There is no vegetable that is off limits, so any, and all, vegetables will put you on the right track to a Mediterranean way of life. Many of the vegetables popular in the Mediterranean regions may be ones that you are already familiar with and use quite regularly, such as tomatoes, spinach, bell peppers, peas, and potatoes. Others may be new to you, such as eggplant, arugula, grape leaves, and artichokes.

TO YOUR HEALTH

The simplest preparation—sautéing your vegetables in olive oil with a few herbs and spices—will guarantee they are never tasteless or boring! Take peas, for example: when sautéed in olive oil with scallions and fresh tomatoes, you have the perfect Mediterranean vegetable dish. So easy and so tasty! (See Chapter 21 for more side dish recipes.)

Healthy Benefits

It's impossible to argue the fact that vegetables are good for you. The vitamins, minerals, antioxidants, phytonutrients, and fiber that vegetables contribute to our daily diet undoubtedly lead to better health. Eating more vegetables as part of an overall healthy diet has been shown to reduce the risk of stroke, heart disease, hypertension, type 2 diabetes, and many types of cancers including stomach, colon, and lung cancers. With their high content of insoluble fibers, they may also lower the risk for diverticulosis, a condition of the large intestines (see Chapter 15 for more information).

When you add more vegetables to your lunch box, dinner plate, and snack time, you are increasing essential nutrients that your body uses to help protect it from disease and maintain its normal function. In addition, adding more vegetables can fill you up, leaving less room for junk foods and other foods with loads of calories, sugar, and fat. This equals weight loss and better maintenance of a healthy weight.

Nutritional Properties of Vegetables

Vegetables are a powerhouse when it comes to nutritional content. Most vegetables are naturally low in calories, fat, and sodium. As an added bonus, they contain no cholesterol, saturated fat, or trans fat. Vegetables provide vitamins, minerals, antioxidants, and phytonutrients such as flavonoids, carotenoids, and indoles. Vegetables also provide the all-important dietary fiber, both soluble and insoluble. Brightly colored vegetables, especially dark green, yellow, orange, and red, are particularly rich in phytonutrients and antioxidants. According to experts, the more brightly colored a vegetable is, the more protective benefits it provides.

Most veggies are major sources of potassium, folate, and two powerful antioxidants: vitamin A and vitamin C. In addition, they deliver other essential nutrients including phosphorus, magnesium, calcium, selenium, iron, manganese, copper, zinc, and vitamin E. Not all vegetables are created equal. Nutritional content differs, so vary your choices daily—and remember that color counts as well!

GOOD TO KNOW

Vegetables are naturally low in fat and calories; however, adding cream sauces or butter can add loads of unhealthy fat, calories, and cholesterol.

Popular Vegetables of the Mediterranean

Vegetables are an important part of the Mediterranean diet, and the variety of vegetables in this region is abundant. You can always find one, and probably many more, that will please your palate. Many of the vegetables eaten in this area are vegetables you probably already enjoy. Let's look at a few of the more common veggies of the Mediterranean.

Artichokes

Artichokes are a strange-looking vegetable. It's a large thistle-type plant that is native to the Mediterranean regions, but it can also be grown in the United States, primarily in California. When choosing artichokes, look for ones that are dark green, heavy, firm, and have tight leaves. If the leaves appear to be opening, are loose, or are turning brown, the vegetable is probably past its prime. Artichokes are normally available year-round, but the peak season is from March to May. Artichokes should be stored in the refrigerator in a plastic bag, unwashed. Your best bet is to cook artichokes within five days of purchase. You can cook artichokes in many different ways including microwaving, steaming, grilling, boiling, braising, sautéing, and even pressure cooking. Once cooked, cool them completely and cover them; they will keep in the refrigerator for up to a week.

Most people have no idea how easy it is to eat an artichoke. In fact, you don't even have use a knife or fork—it is perfectly proper to use your fingers instead. Once cooked, this vegetable can be enjoyed either hot or cold. The leaves of the vegetable are edible and are the best place to start. You simply pluck a leaf and place it between your front teeth, pulling to get the soft, tender flesh that sits at the bottom of the leaf, then discard the rest.

Once all the leaves are gone, you are at the most popular part of the plant: the artichoke heart. Scoop out the fuzzy choke that guards the heart and what you have remaining is the tender heart of the artichoke. This can be used to dip and eat as is, or it can be used in your favorite recipes, dips, stir-fries, omelets, and more.

Artichokes are chock-full of nutrition and contain no fat, cholesterol, or trans fat. They offer a unique array of nutrients and are a good source of protein. Also included in their nutritional profile are potassium, magnesium, folate, the antioxidant vitamin C, and dietary fiber. In fact, they are fiber-rich, containing a whopping 10 grams of fiber in one large artichoke (120 grams) and approximately 7 grams of fiber in $\frac{1}{2}$ cup of cooked artichoke hearts! This makes them one of the vegetables highest in fiber content. If that's not enough to convince you to try this vegetable, you should know that artichokes also contain an array of health-promoting phytonutrients with anti-oxidant properties including flavonoids (such as quercetin and rutin), anthocyanins, gallic acid, polyphenols, caffeic acid, and silymarin. Those might sound a bit foreign by name, but they are some of the most powerful phytonutrients around.

Eggplant

Eggplants are very popular in Mediterranean, Asian, and Middle Eastern cuisine, and they are growing in popularity in the United States. There are numerous varieties of eggplants available, ranging in color from dark purple (which is probably the most familiar) to red, green, white, and yellow, depending on the specific variety. You might be surprised to know that technically eggplants are a fruit but are generally thought of and prepared as a vegetable. They look much like a squash with a tubular or pear shape and are generally quite large in size. The flesh of the eggplant has a bit of a bland flavor; however, its spongelike texture soaks up the flavor of other foods, herbs, and spices that it's cooked with.

Eggplant is very versatile and great when stuffed with a variety of ingredients or broiled, baked, grilled, or sautéed. They are popularly used as appetizers, substituted for pasta in lasagna dishes, and used in place of meat in parmigiana. You can use them in a sandwich or add them to soups and stews.

Eggplant is available all year long, but its peak season is August through September. Look for eggplants that are shiny with a smooth skin containing no bruises or blemishes. An eggplant should be heavy for its size and have a solid sound when tapped. Smaller eggplants generally are sweeter and more tender with a thinner skin and fewer seeds. To be sure the vegetable is ripe, press the side with your finger; if it doesn't make an indentation, it's not ripe. If it does make an indentation but doesn't bounce back, it's overripe and will most likely be bitter. Choose one that is ripe but not too ripe as you can't store eggplants very long. It is best to use them within a few days of purchasing them or picking them from your garden. Store them in a cool, dry place for a few days; if you have to store them longer, keep them in the refrigerator in a plastic bag. They can be very delicate and can bruise easily so be careful when handling them.

The eggplant is low in calories and fat, rich in fiber, and a good source of potassium, iron, protein, folate, manganese, vitamin K, thiamin, niacin, vitamin B_6, pantothenic acid, magnesium, phosphorus, copper, and vitamins A and C (two powerful antioxidants). In addition to featuring a multitude of vitamins, minerals, and antioxidants, eggplants contain health-protective phytonutrients such as phenolic compounds and flavonoids. With only 20 to 30 calories per 1 cup cubed, this food is very nutrient dense—it has loads of nutrition and very few calories.

> **GOOD TO KNOW**
>
> Eggplants, along with other vegetables such as potatoes, tomatoes, sweet peppers, and chile peppers, are classified as nightshade vegetables. Alkaloids, a specific substance found in these types of vegetables, can compromise joint function in people that are highly sensitive, although effects of food on joint function varies greatly among individuals. Cooking can lower the level of alkaloids by about 40 to 50 percent. However, people with joint problems (such as arthritis) or who are highly sensitive to alkaloids may benefit from avoiding this category of vegetables. You should speak with your doctor before making any decisions.

Zucchini

Zucchini may not seem like an exotic vegetable, but it is one of the more common vegetables of the Mediterranean. It has long been a favorite in the regions of the Mediterranean but is now a popular veggie in the United States. Zucchini is the most popular variety of summer squash and is available year-round. However, those ripened during the summer months are known to be more flavorful, with the peak season being May to August. It has a shape and color similar to the cucumber, and its edible flowers are popular in French and Italian cooking.

Zucchini is quite versatile and can be used as a basis for all types of dishes, including pasta sauces, soups and stews, and main dishes. You can even grate it and sprinkle it on salads and sandwiches or add it to homemade breads and muffins. Zucchini has a high water content, so steaming or cooking it as quickly as possible with very little water is recommended. If you overcook zucchini, you basically end up with mush!

Take care when handling zucchini as they can bruise easily, and choose ones that are smaller, because larger zucchini can be less flavorful and more bitter. Look for a moist stem and a shiny skin free of cuts and/or bruises. Like most other vegetables, zucchini is perishable, so only buy what you need. They are best stored in the refrigerator in a plastic bag, preferably in the crisper drawer, for about five days. Do not wash the vegetable until you are ready to use it. It is best to wash it well before eating and leave the skin on, because this is where the majority of the nutrients are.

This vegetable is fiber-rich and a great source of the antioxidants vitamins A and C. In addition, zucchini delivers folate, potassium, magnesium, copper, riboflavin, manganese, phosphorus, thiamin, and vitamin B_6. It boasts health-promoting phytonutrients called carotenoids, specifically beta-carotene and lutein. With its high water content, zucchini is quite low in calories: there are only about 10 calories in $\frac{1}{2}$ cup raw and 14 calories in the same amount cooked.

> **TO YOUR HEALTH**
>
> Any vegetable is better than no vegetable. Fresh is the preferred choice, but when fresh isn't available, frozen or canned vegetables can be just as nutritious. Look for varieties that are low in sodium and do not contain added sauces.

Alternatives You Can Use

All vegetables count when you are following the Mediterranean diet; it makes no difference whether they started out in the Mediterranean regions or in your own backyard. The key is to include them daily and to eat a variety. Some of these vegetables are likely to be very familiar to you, and you might be surprised to find out just how common they are in the Mediterranean, too. It's a small world, isn't it?

Tomatoes

Tomatoes are one of those vegetables that are just as popular in the United States (and many other countries) as they are in the regions of the Mediterranean. In fact, in the United States, tomatoes are second only to potatoes in amount consumed. Botanically speaking, the tomato is considered a fruit; however, because most of us think of and prepare them as vegetables, and because they are more nutritionally like that of a vegetable, that is how they are more commonly classified. Nothing marks the summer months better than a red, juicy, vine-ripened tomato. There are literally thousands of varieties that vary in shape, color, and size. The most common shapes are the round (such as beefsteak or globe), oval-shaped (such as roma or plum), and the smaller bite-size (such as cherry and grape). The yellow tomatoes tend to be less acidic than their red counterparts.

Although tomatoes are available in your grocery store all year long, the peak season—when the best tasting tomatoes show up—is from July through September. Tomatoes are extremely versatile and can be used in an infinite variety of ways including pizza, sandwiches, ketchup, soups, casseroles, salads, dips, salsa … the list goes on.

Choose tomatoes that are round, full, and heavy for their size. The skin should be tight, not shriveled, and be free from bruises and blemishes. Store your tomatoes in a cool, dark place—preferably with the stem side down—and use them within a few days of purchase. Don't store uncut tomatoes in the refrigerator if you don't have to. Too cold of a temperature will change the texture of the tomato's flesh and cause them to lose flavor. Once the tomato is cut, leftover portions should be covered and refrigerated.

Tomatoes are an excellent source of a variety of nutrients including vitamins C, A, and K. They are a good source of potassium, molybdenum, manganese, fiber, chromium, and thiamin. In addition, they deliver vitamin B_6, folate, copper, niacin, riboflavin, magnesium, iron, pantothenic acid, phosphorus, vitamin E, and even a bit of protein. One of the highlights of tomatoes' nutritional content is the powerful antioxidant lycopene, which gives tomatoes their red color.

Mushrooms

Mushrooms are a type of fungus—but one that we enjoy in so many ways. They are not plants; however, they are often classified as a vegetable because of their similar nutritional value and culinary uses. Mushrooms are considered a vegetable on the USDA's MyPyramid as well as on the Mediterranean Diet Pyramid. Mushrooms have become known as nutritional powerhouses and are popular in the Mediterranean and virtually all around the world. Mushrooms can be found in endless varieties with the most common being portobello, white, shiitake, and enoki.

People enjoy mushrooms not only for their taste but also for their versatility. They can be used as an ingredient for dishes such as pizza, pasta, soups, stews, salads, sandwiches, burgers, wraps, casseroles, stir-fries, meat dishes, vegetable dishes, and more. You can add mushrooms to just about any dish for a nutrition boost. You can even use portobellos in place of meat by grilling them and serving them on a bun as a sandwich.

Choose mushrooms that are firm and have a fresh, smooth appearance. The surface should not appear to be dried out. You can keep mushrooms up to a week if refrigerated. Store them in their original container for optimum freshness and, once opened, store the mushrooms in a porous paper bag to prolong their shelf life. Do not freeze fresh mushrooms, only ones that have been cooked. Cooked mushrooms will last up to a month in the freezer. Be sure to clean mushrooms well, but only right before using them.

Mushrooms have been touted as nature's hidden treasure. They are loaded with a large variety of nutrients associated with good health. Mushrooms are rich in selenium, a mineral that acts as an antioxidant and is critical for strengthening the immune system. They also contain another disease-fighting antioxidant known as ergothioneine. Mushrooms are the only "vegetable" that contains vitamin D. In addition, they provide copper, potassium, and B vitamins (including riboflavin, niacin, and pantothenic acid).

Carrots

What can be more common than the carrot? This popular root vegetable boasts a sweet, crunchy taste that makes them a favorite of adults and children alike. They are versatile and full of nutrition. The carrot was originally cultivated in central Asia and the Middle Eastern countries.

Carrots can be enjoyed both raw and cooked. Always wash carrots by gently scrubbing them right before eating. They should also be peeled, especially if they're not organically grown. Carrots can be used in many ways; you can add them to salads, soups, casseroles, stews, breads, and muffins. You can use them as a side dish (on their own or mixed with other veggies) or as a quick and healthy snack.

Choose carrots that are firm, smooth, relatively straight, and bright in color. Carrots are a hardy vegetable and will keep longer than others if stored properly. The trick with carrots is to try to minimize the amount of moisture they lose. Store them in the coolest part of the refrigerator in a plastic bag or airtight container. You should be able to keep them for about two weeks. If you purchase carrots with the greens attached, be sure to cut them off before storing.

Carrots are an excellent source of phytonutrients especially beta-carotene, which possess antioxidant properties and comes from the carotenoid group. This is where carrots get their deep orange color. In fact, they contain more beta-carotene than any other vegetable. Ever hear that carrots can help you see better? Well, here's why: beta-carotene helps to protect vision, especially night vision. In addition this phyto-nutrient can be converted into vitamin A in our liver. Carrots are also high in fiber and supply manganese; niacin; potassium; and vitamins A, B_6, K, and C.

HEALTHY MORSELS

Prepackaged baby carrots can be a great way to keep carrots available for snacking or to use in your favorite recipes. Baby carrots are not babies at all, but rather mature carrots that have been whittled and peeled down to a smaller, more convenient size.

Going for the Super Greens

Chances are your salads are comprised of iceberg lettuce (a salad green that is much less nutritious than its more colorful counterparts) and a few fresh veggies. Maybe a little cheese, some croutons—can't forget the ranch dressing. There is a better way! To make your salads healthier and give them that Mediterranean flair, start the base of your salad with dark green leafy vegetables. Then top them with any vegetable or fruit you wish, beans or nuts, and a wonderful olive oil–based salad dressing. Now you have a salad that you can be proud of!

Many of us don't consume the two to three cups of dark green leafy vegetables recommended by the USDA's MyPyramid (see Chapter 3), yet the Mediterranean diet highly emphasizes these super foods. Dark green leafy vegetables are "super" because they are loaded with a bonanza of essential nutrients including, but not limited to, calcium; iron; folate; potassium; antioxidants (including vitamins A and C); and vita-mins D, E, and K. Furthermore, they are very low in fat and calories and are great sources of fiber. Research suggests that the phytonutrients found in greens may help to prevent certain types of cancer as well as promote heart health.

There is a vast variety of greens that can boost your diet to Mediterranean greatness and can spice up any salad or dish: arugula, kale, spinach, romaine, Swiss chard, mustard greens, and even dandelion greens, just to name a few. Greens can be used in a variety of ways: in salads, sautéed in olive oil as a side dish, or added to soups, side dishes, stir-fries, sandwiches, and other favorite recipes. They can also be used as a wrap with your favorite fillings. On your next shopping trip, choose greens that are fresh with a deep green color. Look for tender, brightly colored leaves with few wilted or yellowed leaves. Always wash greens thoroughly before using and store them in the refrigerator, unwashed in a plastic bag, for up to three days.

TO YOUR HEALTH

Many greens contain fat-soluble vitamins such as vitamins A, D, E, and K. Fat-soluble vitamins require a bit of healthy dietary fat in order to be absorbed into the body, so make sure to add a bit of olive oil to your greens to ensure your body absorbs all of the vitamins it needs.

Here is some information to help rev up your knowledge and intake of nutritious greens:

- Arugula has a spicy, peppery taste. It is rich in vitamins A and C and calcium, and it's extremely low in calories. It can be eaten raw; however, with its strong flavor, is usually best when mixed with milder greens. It can be cooked as well and is popular in salads, stir-fries, soups, and pasta sauces.

- Kale has a slightly bitter flavor and belongs to the group of vegetables that includes collards, cabbage, and Brussels sprouts. It is rich in vitamins A, B_6, C, and K and is a good source of fiber, copper, manganese, calcium, and potassium. Kale is tasty when added to soups, stir-fries, pasta, and sauces. You can even try it as a pizza topping!

- Spinach is a popular green with a sweet yet bitter flavor. It is one of the most nutritious greens, providing an excellent source of manganese, folate, magnesium, iron, riboflavin, calcium, potassium, and vitamins A, B_6, C, and K. Spinach contains at least 13 different types of health-promoting flavonoid compounds (phytonutrients). It can be eaten raw in salads, cooked as a side dish, or added to your favorite recipes like lasagna or pasta. As with other greens, it is quite low in calories.

- Romaine is a popular salad green with a crisp texture. Although it is extremely low in calories and has a high water content, it is actually quite nutritious. Romaine lettuce is an excellent source of folate, manganese, chromium, and vitamins A and C. Additionally it is a good source of fiber, thiamin, riboflavin, potassium, iron, molybdenum, and phosphorus. Start your next salad with romaine instead of iceberg lettuce!

- Swiss chard is very similar to spinach in taste; it also has a bit of a bitter flavor. It's rich in vitamins A, B_6, C, E, and K as well as potassium, magnesium, manganese, iron, and fiber. Additionally it is a good source of copper, calcium, thiamin, riboflavin, folate, zinc, niacin, and protein. It is very tasty whether eaten raw in salads or cooked. It can be tossed into pasta or used as a wrap for your favorite fillings, in omelets, or in place of spinach in dishes like lasagna.

- Mustard greens taste much like arugula with a spicy, peppery flavor. This green is jam-packed with nutrients and phytonutrients including folate, calcium, manganese, and vitamins A, C, K, and E. Mustard greens are delicious in salads, sautéed, added to pasta, or served with beans and rice.

- Dandelion greens are a quick-cooking green with a bitter but tangy flavor. These greens are a great source of calcium, iron, potassium, and vitamins A and K. They are best when used in a salad or on a sandwich, sautéed with other vegetables, or steamed.

HEALTHY MORSELS

Should you always choose organic, locally grown produce? Recommendations for the Mediterranean diet do emphasize locally grown foods, and in a perfect world, we would all enjoy fresh, local, organic produce. But in the real world, it's not always available, or it may be a bit more than your budget allows, so do the best you can. Shop local markets if possible, or at least look for locally grown produce in your neighborhood grocery store. If your choice is organic, all the better. If neither is possible and the best you can do is produce from your supermarket, then that will work. The important thing is that you are including more fruits and vegetables in your daily diet.

Tips for Vegging Out

It's not hard to add more vegetables to your diet, and it will be worth your effort in the long run. Experts suggest that you consume at least five to nine total servings of fruits and vegetables every day. By adding more veggies to your daily diet, you will be reaping the benefits that all those vegetables have to offer. On the Mediterranean diet you will be limiting some foods that you might be used to eating, so try to eat a variety of vegetables that will please your palate—that way, you won't miss what you need to cut out. Here are some tips to help sneak those vegetables into your daily routine:

- Always keep fresh veggies in the refrigerator. Having them cleaned and ready to eat makes it easier to grab as a healthy snack.

- Keep an assortment of bagged vegetables in the freezer so you can easily add them to soups, side dishes, or casseroles when you don't have fresh on hand.

- Add veggies by being creative with your cooking. Add vegetables—or extra vegetables—to sauces, soups, side dishes, casseroles, salads, and pastas. You can never have too many vegetables!

- Use vegetable purées as pasta toppers or as a base for soups and sauces. You can even use a spicy vegetable purée to spread on breads, crackers, or tortillas or as a dip with raw veggies.

- Spice up your morning omelet or scrambled eggs with mushrooms, onions, red peppers, grated zucchini, spinach, or chopped broccoli. Veggies aren't just for dinner anymore!

- Try a vegetable sandwich for lunch wrapped in your favorite tortilla or wrap.

- Fill half of your dinner plate with vegetables.

- Serve soup, chili, stew, pasta, or rice in a scooped-out whole tomato or pepper—and be sure to eat the bowl!

- Add chopped spinach, kale, or other greens to stews, soups, or casseroles. You can even sneak in shredded carrots or zucchini.

- Make it a point to serve a salad full of dark green leafy vegetables with every dinner.

- Make it a goal to try a new vegetable every week, whether it's a side dish or part of a new recipe.

The Least You Need to Know

- Vegetables are one of the foundations of the Mediterranean Diet Pyramid.
- Eating more vegetables as part of a healthy diet has been shown to reduce the risk of stroke, heart disease, hypertension, many types of cancers, type 2 diabetes, and possibly diverticulosis.
- Vegetables are loaded with disease-fighting and health-promoting vitamins, minerals, antioxidants, phytonutrients, and fiber.
- Popular vegetables of the Mediterranean include artichokes, eggplant, and zucchini. However, any vegetable will do as long as you are consuming enough and getting a variety each day.
- The Mediterranean diet emphasizes the use of dark green leafy vegetables. The USDA's MyPyramid recommends adding at least two to three cups daily.
- Getting enough vegetables daily does not need to be difficult, but it does take a little planning and preparation.

Fantastic Seafood

In This Chapter

- Connecting seafood to the Mediterranean diet
- An ocean of health benefits
- What the experts say
- A few common varieties
- Looking at the issues
- Adding more seafood to your diet

People of the Mediterranean have long known something that we are just starting to realize: seafood has tremendous nutritional health benefits. Perhaps you don't think you like fish. However, just as with vegetables, there may be more kinds that you can eat than you might think. There is a vast assortment of fish and shellfish, and they have all different tastes and textures to please even the pickiest of palates. The key is to give them a try!

Connection to the Mediterranean Diet

The Mediterranean diet is a plant-based eating style; however, it is not without its healthy protein sources. It is not surprising, being that the Mediterranean regions are surrounded by water, that one of the recommended and popular protein sources is fish and shellfish. This protein source is readily available to people of the Mediterranean. The seafood group includes everything from salmon to sardines to squid—and many more.

One of the key ideas of the Mediterranean diet is eating more fish and less meat. Seafood is one step up from the plant group on the Mediterranean Diet Pyramid (see Chapter 3). The recommendation of the Mediterranean Diet Pyramid is to eat small to moderate amounts of fish and shellfish at least two times per week.

Healthy Benefits

We know that the health benefits of the Mediterranean diet do not come from just one group of foods but from a combination of healthy foods. Seafood is one piece of that puzzle. Most seafood is low in total fat, but the fat that fish and shellfish does contain is mostly omega-3 fatty acids, better known as the "good" fats. These essential fatty acids protect your heart, decreasing your risk for heart disease. They cannot be produced by our bodies; therefore, we must get them from the foods we eat.

Research has shown that the omega-3 fatty acids in seafood may decrease the risk of sudden death due to arrhythmias (abnormal heartbeats). These fats also help to decrease triglyceride levels. In addition, eating seafood and omega-3 fatty acids have been associated with a lower risk of Alzheimer's disease and stroke. Other health benefits include strengthening the immune system; providing anti-inflammatory properties; relieving joint pain; improving skin and hair condition; improving circulation (and therefore possibly helping to lower blood pressure); and helping the development of the baby's brain, nerves, and eyesight during pregnancy. Eating seafood may even help to reduce the symptoms of depression, anxiety, and attention deficit hyperactivity disorder (ADHD). The bottom line is that seafood is good and good for you—so eat more fish and shellfish!

HEALTHY MORSELS

Ever hear the phrase "fish is brain food"? Fish is linked with healthy brain function, including reducing the decline of cognitive function associated with aging.

The Experts Agree

Still not convinced that seafood needs to be a part of your weekly diet? Experts seem to recommend fish and shellfish across the board. Not only does the Mediterranean diet encourage the consumption of fish, but so do other reputable organizations and sources:

- The American Heart Association (AHA) recommends including at least two servings (about 4 ounces cooked) of fish per week. The AHA recommends eating more fatty fish like salmon, mackerel, herring, lake trout, sardines, and albacore tuna (fresh or canned).

- The Dietary Guidelines for Americans recommends two servings of fish (preferably high in omega-3 fatty acids) per week.

- The American Dietetic Association (ADA) and the Dietitians of Canada recommends two servings of fish per week, preferably fatty fish.

- The American Diabetes Association recommends two or more servings of fish per week (with the exception of commercially fried fish fillets).

- The National Cholesterol Education Program recommends that people choose fish more often.

- The National Academies (Institute of Medicine) state that seafood is part of a healthy diet and can be substituted for other protein sources that are higher in saturated fat.

Nutritional Properties of Seafood

Seafood is low in calories and low in total fat—including the unhealthy saturated fat—with most being low in cholesterol as well. This makes it a great source of high-quality protein and a much better source of protein than animal sources. On average, depending on the type, fish contains about 22 grams of protein per 3.5-ounce cooked serving, or about 6 grams per ounce.

All seafood contains long-chain polyunsaturated omega-3 fatty acids specifically called eicosapentaenoic acid (EPA) and docosahexaenoic acid (DHA), which are nutrients found almost exclusively in seafood. The content of omega-3 fatty acid varies depending on the type of fish or shellfish with the fattier fish being higher:

- The fattiest seafood tend to be cold-water varieties such as salmon, lake trout, mackerel, eel, sardines, herring, fresh albacore tuna, fresh bluefin tuna, orange roughy, and anchovies.

- Leaner seafood includes Pacific halibut, catfish, tilapia, cod, swordfish, flounder, haddock, pollock, shrimp, crabs, crayfish, squid, octopus, oysters, sea bass, and clams.

We know that most seafood is loaded with omega-3 fatty acids, but it doesn't end there. Fish is filled with a variety of essential vitamins and minerals. It's a good source of B vitamins, and fattier fish are a good source of vitamins A and D. Many fish are also a natural source of calcium, phosphorus, iron, potassium, zinc, magnesium, and copper.

> **TO YOUR HEALTH**
>
> Recommended intakes of DHA and EPA have not yet been established by the FDA; however, the American Dietetic Association (ADA) and Dietitians of Canada not only recommend two servings of fatty fish per week but, in addition, 500 mg combined of EPA and DHA per day. Following recommendations by the ADA and the Mediterranean diet and consuming about 8 ounces of cooked fatty fish per week will provide approximately 500 mg of EPA and DHA per day.

Shrimp and a select variety of other seafood often get a bad rap for being too high in cholesterol. However, while the amount of cholesterol you eat is definitely important, there are other factors to consider. These types of seafood may contain moderate amounts of cholesterol, but they are also low in total fat and saturated fat. If you are consuming other foods on the Mediterranean diet that are low in cholesterol, saturated fat, and trans fat (both which can raise blood cholesterol levels), eating shrimp or other seafood higher in cholesterol is fine in moderation. How you cook the shrimp or seafood also counts, so deep-fried or swimming in butter is out. Other seafood higher in cholesterol includes squid, octopus, crayfish, clams, crab, oysters, scallops, and lobster. If you have high cholesterol and are concerned about your seafood selections, speak with your doctor or a registered dietitian.

Selecting Seafood

The more confident you are when shopping for seafood, the more likely you will be to purchase and consume it. To get started, you should know that the category of seafood includes finfish such as salmon, tilapia, and flounder as well as shellfish such as shrimp, clams, and oysters. Follow a few of these helpful tips when shopping for seafood to ensure you purchase high-quality, safe seafood that will fit your personal needs and preferences:

- Always buy fresh or frozen seafood from a reputable source.
- Check that the seafood at the fish counter is properly iced, well refrigerated, and kept in a clean display case.

- Choose the fish that is best for your recipe. Lean fish is best for baking, poaching, and microwaving, while fattier fish tends to do better when grilling and roasting, because it won't dry out as quickly.

- Peak-quality finfish should be firm to the touch and have stiff fins and scales that are tight to the skin. The skin should be moist and shiny and not dry and dull.

- If fish has a strong fishy or sour smell, it's not fresh. Fresh fish should have a mild, fresh, and oceanlike odor.

- If you're buying a whole fish, look at the eyes. If the fish is fresh, the eyes are bright, clear, and protruding (as opposed to dull, hazy, and sunken in). Peak-quality shellfish are generally sold live. Unless they are frozen, canned, or cooked, lobsters, crabs, and crayfish should be living when sold. Clams, mussels, and oysters must be sold live if they are still in their shells. If their shells are removed, they should have a mild, fresh smell.

- If fish or shellfish is frozen, it should be free from freezer burn with no drying or discoloration, mild in odor, and free from ice crystals. Look for any signs of thawing and refreezing, such as freezer burn.

- Choose cooked shrimp with pink to reddish shells. For other crustaceans, the shells should be bright red.

- Stay away from cooked seafood that is displayed alongside raw seafood to avoid cross-contamination.

- Don't purchase seafood that is more than one or two days old, and avoid it if it has been in a display case for extended periods, even if on ice. If you don't know, don't be afraid to ask when the fish came in. The fresher it is, the better it will taste.

- If there isn't fresh fish available, buying fish or shellfish that has been frozen at sea is your next best option. You are better off buying salmon or other fish that has been frozen and then recently thawed than to buy fresh fish that has been sitting, unfrozen, for several days.

- The easiest preparation option is to purchase fillets or steaks, both of which are ready to cook.

Popular Seafood Choices of the Mediterranean

Seafood is prominent in many Mediterranean dishes and recipes. Some of the more popular choices may be varieties you already prepare and enjoy. Many of the common seafood included on the Mediterranean diet include fattier fish, which are higher in omega-3 fatty acids. However, there are also leaner choices, and it's best to consume a variety. According to the Mediterranean Diet Pyramid, some common varieties include abalone, cockles, clams, crab, eel, flounder, lobster, mackerel, mussels, octopus, oysters, salmon, sardines, sea bass, shrimp, squid, tilapia, tuna, whelk, and yellowtail. Keep in mind that any type of fish or seafood will do when it comes to following the Mediterranean diet, but choose fattier fish more often—at least once per week.

Salmon

Just as it is in the United States, salmon is one of the more common finfish in the Mediterranean regions. Salmon is a fish that even people who don't care for fish tend to favor. These fish are classified as either Pacific or Atlantic depending on where they're caught. There is one type of Atlantic salmon; however, there are five types of Pacific salmon: Chinook (or king), sockeye, coho, pink, and chum. They range in color from pink to red to orange, and some are fattier than others depending on the variety, where they are caught, and whether they are wild or farm-raised. Salmon is low in mercury content and has a high nutritional content. It's an excellent source of protein and is low in calories and saturated fat. Salmon is a great source of omega-3 fatty acids and has the perfect health-supportive ratio of omega-3 to omega-6 fatty acids. Omega-6 fatty acids are another group of essential fatty acids necessary for health. However, we don't have as much of a problem getting them in our diets as we do with omega-3 fatty acids (see Chapter 14). Salmon is a good source of vitamin D; in fact, a 4-ounce serving of wild salmon provides all the vitamin D you need for the day—there aren't too many foods that can make that claim. That same serving of fish contains vitamins B_6 and B_{12}, niacin, selenium, phosphorus, and magnesium.

You can buy salmon frozen, fresh, canned, or smoked. Frozen salmon can taste great because it is usually flash-frozen soon after being caught. Look for fish that is wrapped well and free of ice crystals, visible blood, and discoloration on the skin and flesh. Fresh salmon can be purchased whole or in the form of steaks or fillets. Don't buy fresh salmon if it has a strong fishy smell. Canned salmon is almost always wild and contains a significant amount of calcium because there are small but edible bones of the fish included. Smoked salmon is a method used to preserve the fish but it can be high in sodium as well as price. Due to salmon's fat content, it holds up well to many different cooking methods without drying out. It is thick enough to throw on the grill and fatty enough to bake, poach, broil, or pan-fry. When baking or grilling, it should cook just until it flakes to keep it from drying out. Salmon is a versatile fish and pairs well with a wide variety of flavors. It is not a delicate fish, so it does well with sauces, rubs, herbs, and marinades.

Here are a few ideas:

- Put a salmon fillet on a piece of aluminum foil. Top it with capers, crushed garlic, and a bit of lemon juice. Drizzle a small amount of olive oil and white wine on top. Fold up the foil so that the edges seal into a packet, and bake it at 350°F for about 15 to 20 minutes or until flaky.

- Poach salmon in an inch of vegetable broth with a little dill. Serve it with a dollop of nonfat plain Greek yogurt.

- Marinate salmon steak in olive oil, honey, and lime juice overnight and cook on the grill until flaky.

- Marinate salmon in extra-virgin olive oil and diced garlic and bake it until flaky.

- Substitute canned salmon for canned tuna in any recipe.

HEALTHY MORSELS

There is a growing controversy about which is best: wild or farmed salmon. Farmed salmon is regulated by the USDA and FDA, but the wild version is regulated by the Environmental Protection Agency, which has much stricter guidelines. Farmed salmon is usually fattier, offering more omega-3 fatty acids; however they also, on average, contain more environmental contaminants (such as PCBs and mercury) because these contaminants are stored in fat. The bottom line is that, whenever possible, you should choose wild over farmed salmon. This goes for other fish and shellfish as well. If only farmed salmon is available, the health benefits of the fish may outweigh the risk of the possible contaminants. To help reduce your exposure, trim the skin and visible fat on fish and prepare it by grilling or broiling to help reduce a significant portion of the fat.

Tuna

Tuna is found in the Pacific, Atlantic, and Indian oceans and the Mediterranean Sea. Fresh tuna is frequently enjoyed by coastal populations (like those surrounding the Mediterranean Sea), while canned tuna is the number one consumed fish for Americans. Tuna is one of the fattier types of fish and is higher in omega-3 fatty acids. Tuna comes in several varieties including yellowfin, bluefin, and albacore (also called "white") tuna. Albacore tuna is one of the best fish sources of omega-3 fatty acids.

As with all fresh fish, choose fresh tuna that has no strong fishy odor. Tuna needs to be kept cold and is very perishable. Canned tuna is available in chunks or solid and can be packed in oil, broth, or water. Because most canned versions packed in oil use an oil high in omega-6 fatty acids, and most Americans already consume too many of these fats, it is best to choose ones packed in water or broth.

Besides being a good source of omega-3 fatty acids, tuna is an excellent source of niacin, selenium, and high-quality protein. It's also a very good source of thiamin, vitamin B_6, potassium, phosphorus, and magnesium.

Tuna is a meaty fish and is sold fresh or frozen as steaks or fillets. Tuna is also sold as pieces as in the canned version. If you haven't tried fresh tuna, you don't know what you're missing. The fresh version is much higher in omega-3 fatty acids and other nutrients, is delicious, and can be prepared in a variety of ways. Because the Mediterranean diet is all about eating fewer processed foods, fresh tuna is clearly the way to go when possible.

Here are a few ideas:

- Try tuna steaks on the grill. Marinate it first with extra-virgin olive oil, lemon juice, and garlic.

- Replace canned tuna with freshly cooked tuna in your tuna salad recipes or in other salads.

- Cut tuna steaks or fillets into chunks and place on skewer with mushrooms, onions, tomatoes, peppers, or other vegetables. Marinate and cook on the grill.

- Roast tuna with paprika, chopped tomato, garlic, onion, and sweet peppers in the oven.

- Season tuna with a little salt and pepper or your favorite herbs and spices, then grill and serve over fresh ripe figs.

Sardines

Sardines are tiny fish that can be found on coasts all over the world, including near many Mediterranean regions. In fact, sardines were named after an island of the Mediterranean called Sardinia, where they were once quite abundant. There are more then 20 different species of small fish that are actually sold as sardines around the world. Canned sardines in most supermarkets are usually small sprat or herring fish but once canned are considered and labeled as sardines. Pilchard is known as the "true" sardine.

Sardines are among the healthiest choices when it comes to fish and are delicious and inexpensive. Sardines can be purchased fresh or canned; however, fresh sardines will not keep long (only a day or two) and they don't freeze well, so use them quickly.

Choose whole sardines that have a clean smell, are firm to the touch, and have bright eyes. Sardines packed in olive oil are the preferred canned form (as opposed to those canned in soybean oil or other oils) but they also come packed in water as well as sauces such as tomato or mustard. Always check the can for an expiration date to ensure freshness.

Sardines might be tiny but they provide a powerful punch of omega-3 fatty acids. They are also low in contaminants such as mercury because they are so small and so low on the food chain. They feed on organisms such as algae and therefore do not ingest the heavy metals, like mercury, that other fish do. They are an excellent source of iron, vitamin B_{12}, and tryptophan. They also provide protein, calcium, phosphorus, selenium, niacin, and vitamin D. In fact, the canned variety, which usually includes soft, edible bones, has about 35 percent of the recommended daily value for calcium. If bones are removed, so is much of the calcium.

You can cook and serve sardines in a variety of tasty ways. Here are a few ideas:

- Serve canned sardines broiled on whole-wheat toast for a simple, classic appetizer.

- Combine skinless, boneless sardines with half of a diced avocado. Drizzle with Worcestershire sauce, black pepper, and a dash of olive oil for the perfect healthy snack.

- Wrap fresh sardines in grape or fig leaves and grill with olive oil and lemon.

- Sprinkle sardines with lemon juice, extra-virgin olive oil, and a touch of garlic or your favorite herb or spice.

- Try combining sardines with chopped onion, olives, chopped tomatoes, or fennel.

Cooking Up Fish

The best way to enjoy fish is baked, grilled, broiled, poached, stir-fried, sautéed—basically, any way that isn't deep-fried. Avoid heavily battered fried fish as well as highly processed fish products like fish sticks. Choose low-fat, low-sodium seasonings such as herbs, spices, lemon juice, or other flavorings when cooking and serving seafood. Extra-virgin olive oil always makes a good base for marinades. Fish is generally a quick-cooking food; if thawed, it only needs to cook about 10 minutes for every inch of thickness. To check if fish is done, use a knife to cut into the thickest part and pull it aside. If it begins to flake, it is probably done. Another clue is that once fish becomes opaque, it is ready to eat. Once you remove the fish from the heat, let it stand for a few minutes to finish the cooking process.

TO YOUR HEALTH

If you are not a fish lover, get creative with recipes to keep it interesting and tasting great. Check out the recipes in Part 4 for some delicious ideas.

A Few Issues

There always seem to be a few issues, no matter what food you are talking about and seafood is no exception. One common issue when it comes to fish and shellfish is whether taking a fish oil supplement can take the place of eating seafood. Another concern is whether there is too much mercury, or other contaminants, in fish to deem it safe.

Using Fish Oil Supplements

Maybe you are not a fish lover but you do love the idea of all the essential nutrients, especially those omega-3 fatty acids, which fish provides. There has been an ongoing controversy about fish oil supplements and whether they are as beneficial as eating fish. Fish oil supplements usually come in the form of capsules and most contain both DHA and EPA, two forms of omega-3 fatty acids found in fish, especially fatty fish.

The American Heart Association (AHA) says that it is preferable to increase your consumption of omega-3 fatty acids through foods; however, people with coronary artery disease and/or high triglycerides may not be able to consume enough omega-3 fats by diet alone. They suggest, for these people, to speak with their doctors about the use of fish oil supplements. The position of the American Dietetic Association (ADA) on nutritional supplements is that they can help some individuals meet their individual nutrient needs if their diet is inadequate due to extenuating circumstances. They recommend a food-based approach for the intake of fatty acids such as omega-3s but for individuals who do not eat fish, other options can be pursued such as foods fortified with these fatty acids or even supplements.

The bottom line? Currently there is no one answer that fits all. Most experts recommend getting your omega-3 fatty acids from foods, which includes more then just seafood. However, most seem to agree that supplements, in the correct dosage, can be used to "supplement" the diet but not completely take the place of omega-3 containing foods.

If choosing a fish oil supplement, take a good look at the label on the bottle. A supplement may list 1 gram (or 1,000 mg) of fish oil, but that doesn't mean it's all coming from omega-3 fatty acids. The amount of EPA and DHA is the most important component, because these are the true indicators of the amount of heart-healthy omega-3 fatty acids in the supplement. For example, if the label states that the 1,000-mg fish oil supplement contains 250 mg of EPA and 250 mg of DHA, then it has a total of 500 mg of omega-3 fatty acids, not 1,000 mg. In addition, check the label for a 3:2 ratio of either 3 parts EPA to 2 parts DHA or vice-versa. Research suggests that either ratio is optimal for producing heart-healthy benefits.

Fish oil has Generally Recognized As Safe (GRAS) status in the United States. However, currently there is no standard RDA (Recommended Daily Allowance) for EPA and DHA in the form of supplements. The FDA recommends that people do not exceed 3 grams per day of EPA and DHA omega-3 fatty acids, with no more then 2 grams per day in the form of a dietary supplement. Ongoing research points out that it is reasonable for most people to get up to 1,000 mg or 1 gram of EPA and DHA daily.

GOOD TO KNOW

People who take fish oil supplements need to be aware of possible overdosing. Problems such as excessive bleeding can occur in large doses of 3 grams or more. Keep in mind that if you eat fatty fish twice weekly, you may already be getting all or most of what you need.

Use only reputable brands that are pharmaceutical grade, which means it has met freshness and purity standards and often contain a higher potency of EPA and DHA in a single capsule. Because the FDA does not regulate supplements, it's best to look for a supplement that has met purity and freshness standards through third-party testing (such as www.consumerlab.com), which you can find by looking at the label for a certification seal or calling the company's toll-free number. Contaminants such as mercury and PCBs can accumulate in fish oil just as they do in fish, so look for supplements made from purified fish oil. If you decide that fish oil supplements are the way to go, be forewarned: taking more than the recommended dose can increase your risk of bleeding and bruising, which isn't likely to happen from foods.

GOOD TO KNOW

Consult with your health-care provider before taking a fish oil supplement (or any supplement), especially if you have a medical condition, are taking prescription medications, or have food allergies. Always let your doctor know if you are taking fish oil supplements because they inhibit blood clotting, which may cause excessive bleeding for some people.

Mercury Levels

Although seafood is abundantly healthy, balancing its benefits with its concerns about mercury and contaminant levels may leave you a bit confused. Don't give up on fish, though! It is still an excellent choice. You should be knowledgeable about this issue, but it should not keep you from making seafood a part of your diet.

Nearly all fish and shellfish contain traces of mercury; however, for most of us, the risk of mercury in fish is not much of a health concern. The concern is mostly for pregnant women: some fish contain high levels of mercury that could harm an unborn baby or a young child's developing nervous system. For this reason, the FDA and the Environmental Protection Agency advise women who are or may become pregnant, nursing mothers, and young children to avoid some types of fish that are higher in mercury and to eat fish and shellfish that contain lesser amounts of mercury. The advisory states for this population:

- Do not eat shark, swordfish, king mackerel, or tilefish because they contain higher levels of mercury.

- Eat up to 12 ounces (2 average meals) a week of a variety of fish and shellfish that are lower in mercury, such as shrimp, canned light tuna, salmon, pollock, and catfish. Albacore (white) tuna, fresh or canned, has more mercury than canned light tuna; you may eat up to 6 ounces of albacore tuna per week.

- Check local advisories about the safety of fish if caught in local lakes, rivers, and coastal areas. If you cannot find information on local fish, eat up to 6 ounces per week of fish caught from local waters, and do not consume any other fish that week.

- These same recommendations hold true for young children, but they are to be served smaller portions.

The bottom line is that even with these advisories in mind, the AHA's recommendations are to eat two servings of fish per week. At 3 to 4 ounces per serving, that is well below the FDA and Environmental Protection Agency's safe limit of 12 ounces per week. Eating a variety of fish and following the recommendations will ensure that you can still enjoy fish, feel safe, and enjoy all its health benefits.

TO YOUR HEALTH

For more information on this advisory and mercury and contaminant content of fish, go to www.epa.gov/fishadvisories/advice.

Tips for Adding More Fish

Fish might not have been part of your diet before, but now that you know about the health benefits of fish and how easy it can be to prepare, you may have changed your mind. Because following the Mediterranean diet is your ultimate goal, adding these foods is a must. Here are a few ideas to help get you started:

- Ease seafood into your diet by replacing one meat meal per week with one that contains fish or seafood. Work your way up to at least two meals per week.

- Add canned tuna or salmon to your salads to boost the protein and nutrition.

- Prepare your seafood with olive oil, garlic, herbs, and spices to add flavor. Try breading fish with whole-wheat flour and a few breadcrumbs and sautéing it in olive oil.

- Don't forget: it isn't just fish that counts, so include other seafood such as shrimp, crab, lobster, oysters, and mussels.

- Be sure you are buying fresh fish for the best flavor.

- Halibut, fresh tuna, or swordfish steaks marinated and cooked on the grill make a delicious and healthy alternative to red meat.

- Experiment with fish-based soups such as clam chowder or lobster bisque.

- Learn how to cook fish properly. Overcooking fish makes it tough and dry, which hinders the flavor. Remember that fish is cooked when its flesh turns opaque and flakes easily when poked with a fork.

- If you enjoy leaner fish such as tilapia or catfish, consider adding another serving of a fattier fish to your weekly menu to boost your intake of omega-3 fatty acids.

The Least You Need to Know

- Fish and shellfish are a main protein source in the Mediterranean diet.
- Heart-protective omega-3 fatty acids are one of the most important nutrients that seafood provides.
- Fattier, cold-water fish are higher in omega-3 fatty acids.
- Consult your health-care provider before using a fish oil supplement, because they are not a good fit for everyone.
- By following the recommendations of the AHA and Environmental Protection Agency, you can eat fish safely without worrying about ingesting too many contaminants.

Nutty for Nuts, Seeds, and Legumes

In This Chapter

- A good reason to go nutty
- Beans are music to the ear
- How to store and prepare nuts, seeds, and legumes
- Favorite nuts, seeds, and legumes of the Mediterranean
- Go nuts for dessert
- Adding more nuts, seeds, and legumes to your diet

Nuts, seeds, and legumes are plant foods that should not be overlooked. They are all essential additions to a healthy diet. These foods are a category of plants that have pods (or fruits) and include beans, peas, lentils, and peanuts, among others. Nuts are anything with an edible kernel and hard shell. Nuts and legumes are technically seeds, but the seeds we discuss in this chapter are the smaller edible plant seeds that are directly meant for eating rather than for yielding more plants. This group of foods might be small in size, but they're big on nutrition—and a big part of the Mediterranean diet.

Connection to the Mediterranean Diet

Nuts, seeds, and legumes are all included in the plant group, which is the foundation of the Mediterranean Diet Pyramid (see Chapter 3). The pyramid recommends eating an abundance of plant-based foods, which includes legumes, nuts, and seeds, and basing most meals on these plant-based foods. Nuts and seeds are commonly used as a snack in the Mediterranean, and nuts are a popular ingredient in many desserts.

The Mediterranean diet is filled with fabulous dishes using many different varieties of legumes and nuts. A wide variety of these foods are used in the Mediterranean regions including lentils, chickpeas, almonds, hazelnuts, walnuts, fava beans, cannellini beans, pine nuts, sesame seeds, sunflower seeds, and split peas.

Health Benefits of Nuts and Seeds

At one time nuts were given a bad rap for their high fat and calorie content, but now they are known worldwide as a healthy food. Seeds, too, provide a fairly high dose of fat. Both nuts and seeds contain the heart-healthy kind of fat giving them a heart- and health-friendly reputation. Research has found that people who eat nuts on a regular basis have a lower risk for heart disease and sudden cardiac death. Studies have also found that nuts can lower LDL or "bad" cholesterol levels in the blood. The benefits of nuts and seeds are still under the microscope, but more research and results are emerging all the time.

Nuts and seeds may be high in calories due to their fat content; however, because of their nutritional makeup, they can help to reduce hunger by making you feel full and satisfied. Moderation is the key, but nuts and seeds, along with a healthy diet and exercise, may actually help you to lose weight or maintain a healthy weight. The fiber in nuts and seeds help prevent constipation and hemorrhoids. The powerful antioxidants they provide can help to slow the aging process and lower the risk of many age-related health conditions.

In 2003, the FDA approved a health claim on food labels for specific nuts containing less than 4 grams of saturated fat per 50 grams of nuts: almonds, hazelnuts, peanuts, pecans, some pine nuts, pistachios, and walnuts. The claim states, "Scientific evidence suggests but does not prove that eating 1.5 ounces per day of most nuts *[such as name of specific nut]* as part of a diet low in saturated fat and cholesterol may reduce the risk of heart disease."

GOOD TO KNOW

Keep in mind that even though nuts and seeds are healthy, covering them with salt, sugar, or chocolate will cancel out most of their health benefits.

The FDA-approved health claim doesn't mean you should restrict your intake to only these types of nuts. In addition to a variety of nuts, you should include seeds, which may offer the same health benefits. The best approach to using nuts and seeds to your advantage and reaping all of their health benefits is to eat them in moderation and to eat them as a replacement for, not an addition to, foods in your diet that are high in saturated fats and/or trans fats. Nuts and seeds contain quite a bit of fat, and even though most of the fat is a healthy fat, it can still add up to a lot of calories. Stick to just a handful, 1 to 2 ounces, per day. You will get all of the health benefits without getting too many of the calories.

As with most other foods we have discussed, not all nuts and seeds are created equal. They all differ in their nutritional makeup. At the top of the list for heart health are walnuts, almonds, hazelnuts, and pecans. Your best bet is to eat a variety of nuts and seeds.

Health Benefits of Legumes

There are no magical foods, but if you knew all that legumes have to offer, you might consider them almost magical. Legumes are a family of plants whose seeds develop inside pods. They include beans, peas, lentils, peanuts, and soynuts. With their soluble fiber content, legumes can help to lower LDL or "bad" cholesterol levels, thus lowering the risk for heart disease. Soluble bean fiber has a low glycemic index, so it's valuable to diabetics as it helps to slow the absorption of sugar into the blood, helping to control blood sugar levels. The rich source of antioxidants boasted by beans has been linked to lowering the risk for several types of cancer, including colon cancer. A bonus for dieters is that legumes are low in calories; foods, like beans, that have a low glycemic index and are high in fiber can help keep hunger at bay by filling you up, not filling you out. Including beans in your diet on a regular basis can also aid in digestion and normalize bowel function, which can help to prevent constipation and hemorrhoids. Basic legumes supply a load of heart-protective, disease-fighting benefits for very little money, and, in the form of peanuts or soynuts, are as simple as popping a handful into your mouth.

HEALTHY MORSELS

With their nutritional components, legumes, nuts, and seeds make the perfect substitution for vegetarians or for those trying to cut back on meat and saturated fat intake. The USDA's MyPyramid counts ¼ cup of cooked legumes as equivalent to 1 ounce of cooked meat. In addition, ½ ounce of nuts or seeds is equivalent to 1 ounce of meat.

Nutritional Properties of Nuts and Seeds

The Mediterranean diet is filled with healthy fats, but it isn't only the olives and olive oil that provide these fats. You could say they are high-fat foods; however, the fats they do contain are ones you definitely want in your diet. Nuts and seeds provide both monounsaturated and polyunsaturated fats but contain very little saturated fat and no trans fat. Some, such as walnuts, Brazil nuts, flaxseeds, and pumpkin seeds contain omega-3 fatty acids, but they contain a different source than that found in fish. They contain the plant-based source of omega-3 fatty acids known as alpha-linolenic acid (ALA), which can be converted in the body to EPA and DHA, the fatty acids found mostly in fish.

Nuts and seeds contain vitamin E, a powerful antioxidant known for enhancing the immune system, protecting our nervous system, and lowering the risk for heart disease. They are also a great source of vitamin A, phosphorus, potassium, folate, magnesium, copper, selenium, protein, and fiber. Seeds are among the best plant sources of both iron and zinc.

Some nuts and seeds such as cashews, pecans, and walnuts contain plant sterols, a compound found in vegetable oils that can help to lower cholesterol levels. These plant sterols are now being added to many food products (such as margarines), but in some nuts and seeds they are a natural occurrence. Don't leave out phytonutrients in this group of foods, either; they contain a variety of health-promoting phytonutrients, including flavonoids.

Nutritional Properties of Legumes

Legumes are among the most versatile and nutritious foods available. Most are low in fat and contain no cholesterol or trans fats, and some, such as soybeans, navy beans, and kidney beans, contain the plant-based source of the heart-healthy omega-3 fatty acids. They are rich sources of folate, copper, potassium, and magnesium, and most are also a good source of iron and B vitamins. Legumes are a bountiful source of both soluble and insoluble fiber: just 1 cup of legumes can provide as much as 15 grams of fiber. That's half of the daily requirement for most people. As if that weren't enough, legumes are a great source of protein, offering a whopping 15 grams of protein in a 1-cup serving. Soybeans offer even more! While just about all plant-based food offers various health-promoting phytonutrients, the family of legumes is at the top of the list as one of the most phytodense food sources. These include flavonoids, isoflavones, and more. Legumes, especially black, red, and brown beans, are among the richest sources of antioxidants. In addition, like nuts and seeds, legumes offer plant sterols.

TO YOUR HEALTH

Beans are known as the "musical fruit" due to their gas-causing effects. However, if they are soaked in water for at least a few hours before cooking, they will cause less flatulence and, as a bonus, be easier to cook. Canned beans can also reduce gas, as the canning process eliminates some of the gas-producing sugars.

Storing and Preparing Nuts, Seeds, and Legumes

Most nuts and seeds can be eaten raw, but roasting them can help to intensify their flavor. Nuts are sold either shelled or unshelled, and either fresh or, more commonly, dried. Unshelled nuts can be kept for up to a year, and unhulled seeds several months, if stored in a cool, dark, dry place. Shelled nuts and seeds will not keep as long and are more prone to rancidity. They should be kept in an airtight container in the refrigerator and used by their expiration date.

The best part of legumes, besides their star nutritional profile, is they are available year-round, inexpensive, and versatile. The bland taste of beans makes them the perfect sponge to soak up the flavor of any dish. Most can be found dried or canned and have long shelf lives. They are the perfect addition to your pantry to whip up a Mediterranean-style dish in no time. However, a little planning may be needed, as many dried beans are best soaked before cooking. You can always cook beans and freeze them for later use as well.

Popular Nuts and Seeds of the Mediterranean

Nuts and seeds play an important role in the traditional diet of the Mediterranean and throughout the world. There is a large variety of nuts and seeds that are common to the Mediterranean that may be sitting in your pantry already: almonds, cashews, hazelnuts, pine nuts, pistachios, sesame seeds, and walnuts, just to name a few.

Walnuts

Walnuts have one of the highest contents of omega-3 fatty acids of all nuts and seeds, making them a very heart-healthy food. They are a good source of monounsaturated fats, manganese, and copper. Eating walnuts has many potential health benefits including heart health, lowered cholesterol, improved cognitive function, anti-inflammatory benefits, bone health, and even lowered risk for gallstones. Walnuts, along with pecans and chestnuts, have some of the highest antioxidant contents of all tree nuts. Walnuts specifically contain an antioxidant called ellagic acid that helps to support the immune system and may help protect against several types of cancer. Need even more proof? Walnuts contain high levels of the essential amino acid l-arginine, which helps to keep the inner walls of the blood vessels smooth, reduces the risk for hypertension, and helps lower blood pressure.

Walnuts are a delicious way to add a boost of nutrition, flavor, and crunch to any dish, including baked goods, soups, sauces, cooked vegetables, stuffing, stews, and salads. In addition they make a convenient and highly nutritious snack.

HEALTHY MORSELS

The FDA has approved a health claim for walnuts that states, "Supportive but not conclusive research shows that eating 1.5 ounces per day of walnuts, as part of a low saturated fat and low cholesterol diet and not resulting in increased caloric intake, may reduce the risk of coronary heart disease."

Pine Nuts

Pine nuts are a major part of the cuisine throughout the Middle East and Mediterranean regions. This particular nut is especially high in protein, with just 1 ounce of pine nuts yielding about 4 grams of protein. This makes them a great choice for a vegetarian diet. Like walnuts, they, too, are a good source of the amino acid l-arginine, which helps to protect the heart. Pine nuts are high in monounsaturated fats and low in saturated fat. They have the highest concentration of a specific monounsaturated fat called oleic acid that helps to lower triglyceride levels in the body. They are a good source of fiber and iron and an excellent source of magnesium. In addition, they contain copper; zinc; thiamin; riboflavin; potassium; manganese; selenium; folate; niacin; and vitamins A, B_6, E, and K. Pine nuts supply plenty of health-promoting antioxidants and phytonutrients as well.

Pine nuts have a sweet, buttery flavor and delicate texture. They are especially good in salads and can be used on desserts. They are best known for their use in pesto, a sauce traditionally made from pine nuts, fresh basil, garlic, grated cheese, and olive oil (see recipe in Chapter 17). They make a perfect on-the-go snack and can be eaten raw or lightly toasted, which enhances their flavor. Roasting them in the oven with a bit of olive oil adds even more heart-healthy monounsaturated fats. Once they are shelled, pine nuts tend to go rancid quickly and should be stored in the refrigerator to prolong their shelf life and maintain their nutritional content.

Sesame Seeds

Sesame seeds are popular in many Middle Eastern dishes. They add a nutty taste and are available in a variety of colors including brown, red, black, yellow, and ivory. These seeds are a very good source of copper, manganese, magnesium, calcium, iron, phosphorus, thiamin, and zinc. Sesame seeds are a good source of fiber and healthy monounsaturated fats. They contain a phytoestrogen known as lignan that is an antioxidant and may have anticancer effects. In addition, they contain a substance called phytosterols, which may help to block cholesterol production. Sesame seeds may also lower cholesterol levels and blood pressure, fight cancer, provide relief from rheumatoid arthritis, support bone health and vascular and respiratory health, and boost the body's antioxidant capacity. With the combination of nutrients that sesame seeds contain and the possible health benefits, you have plenty of reasons to add them to your diet.

Sesame seeds with their shells should be stored in an airtight container in a cool, dark, dry place. Once the seeds are hulled, like many other nuts and seeds, they are more prone to rancidity and should be stored in the refrigerator or freezer.

The nutty flavor of sesame seeds can add a special touch to even the most basic dish. They are perfect in salads, dressings, vegetables, rice dishes, stir-fries, and baked goods such as breads and muffins. Sesame seeds are the main ingredient in tahini (sesame seed paste) and in the Middle Eastern treat halvah. Tahini can be spread on breads and drizzled with honey for a sweet treat. Tahini is also used in hummus.

Popular Legumes of the Mediterranean

Because the Mediterranean diet is mostly a plant-based eating style, legumes play a significant role. They are filling, full of protein and other essential nutrients, and inexpensive and versatile, thus they make the perfect replacement for red meats and other high-fat meats. Legumes encompass a wide variety of beans, lentils, peanuts, and peas. Legumes such as cannellini beans, chickpeas, fava beans, kidney beans, green beans, lentils, split peas, and peanuts are common to the Mediterranean.

Lentils

Lentils are a staple in Middle Eastern cuisine and in dishes throughout the world. Compared to other dried legumes, lentils are quick and easy to prepare. Lentils tend to absorb the flavors from the foods and seasonings they are cooked and served with. They are sold either whole or split and come in red, brown, and green varieties. The most commonly sold lentil in grocery stores is the brown variety, but green and red lentils can usually be found at specialty food stores. Canned lentils can be just as nutritionally loaded as those you cook yourself; however, you should look for ones without added sodium.

Lentils may be small, but don't let that fool you. They are packed with plenty of nutrition. Lentils are rich in protein without all of the fat and cholesterol of animal sources, making them a common meat substitute in vegetarian dishes. Lentils are excellent sources of folate and molybdenum and are a good source of soluble and insoluble fiber, manganese, iron, phosphorus, copper, thiamin, and potassium. Lentils also provide various phytonutrients that have an antioxidant effect and can help to protect from diseases such as cancer. If you were to look at a chart of fiber in foods, you would discover that legumes like lentils lead the pack. The soluble fiber that lentils contain can lower cholesterol and the risk for heart disease as well as help to control blood sugar in diabetics. The insoluble fiber that lentils provide may help to prevent constipation and digestive disorders.

You should store lentils in an airtight container in a cool, dry, dark place for up to 12 months. Lentils need no presoaking as other legumes do and cook quickly. Cooked lentils can be stored in the refrigerator in a covered container for about three days. Cooked lentils combine well with salads, pastas, rice dishes, cooked vegetables, soups, and stews.

Peanuts

Synonymous with the ballpark and the circus, peanuts are a big part of American culture, but they are also a very common legume in the Mediterranean regions. Don't let the word *nut* in the name of this food fool you; technically, peanuts are a legume, although they have a nutrient profile closer to that of a nut.

Like nuts and unlike most legumes, peanuts are high in the polyunsaturated fats and the heart-healthy monounsaturated fats that are emphasized in the Mediterranean. The type of monounsaturated fats found in peanuts is oleic acid, which is also found in olive oil. Peanuts contain no cholesterol or trans fats, both of which raise cholesterol levels and your risk for heart disease and stroke. Peanuts are a terrific source of protein, providing about 7 grams in just 1 ounce of raw peanuts. In addition, peanuts are a good source of fiber and other essential nutrients including vitamin E, niacin, folate, copper, riboflavin, phosphorus, magnesium, and manganese. Just 1 ounce of peanuts will provide you with 16 percent of your daily needs for vitamin E, which has been shown to act as an antioxidant reducing the risk for heart disease.

Peanuts are rich in health-promoting phytonutrients including resveratrol, which falls into the polyphenol group. This phytonutrient is also found in grape skins, red wine, and grape juice and is thought to be one of the compounds responsible for many of the health benefits associated with the Mediterranean diet. Peanuts' nutritional components can help reduce your risk for heart disease, stroke, cancer, gallstones, Alzheimer's disease, and cognitive decline.

Peanuts come raw or roasted, shelled or unshelled. In fact, roasting peanuts is said to optimize their antioxidant content. It's important to store shelled peanuts, especially raw ones, in a tightly sealed container in the refrigerator or freezer because heat, humidity, and light can all cause rancidity. They will keep this way for up to three months in the refrigerator and six months in the freezer. Unshelled peanuts should be kept in a cool, dark place; keeping them in the refrigerator will extend their shelf life to about nine months.

Peanuts, especially raw ones, need to be stored correctly; in the wrong environment, they can grow a highly dangerous fungus called aflatoxin, which is a known carcinogen. Throw away peanuts that are discolored, shriveled, or moldy.

Peanut butter is another peanut choice; however, it lacks the fiber of whole peanuts and may include salt, sugar, and trans fats that are added during processing. Flavored and roasted peanuts can also be high in sodium.

Peanuts are versatile and can be used in a number of ways. They are great sprinkled on tossed salads, added to sautéed chicken and vegetables, sprinkled on yogurt, mixed with raisins and other dried fruit, or eaten plain as a snack.

> **TO YOUR HEALTH**
>
> Although nuts are a healthy food source, it's important to realize that peanuts and tree nuts are among the top foods linked to allergic reactions. Tree nuts include almonds, cashews, walnuts, pecans, pistachios, Brazil nuts, hazelnuts, and chestnuts. People with allergies to peanuts and tree nuts must be diligent about reading food labels, asking questions, and being on the lookout for hidden ingredients so that they avoid nuts at all costs.

Cannellini Beans

The variety of beans is endless, but the cannellini bean, also known as the white kidney bean or fazolia bean, is a favorite in the Mediterranean regions. It is known for its smooth texture and nutty flavor and is commonly found in minestrone soup or bean salads. These white kidney beans hold up well during cooking and readily absorb flavors of foods, herbs, and spices they are cooked with.

Cannellini beans are low in calories and fat and are an excellent source of fiber, helping to lower cholesterol, promote heart health, and control blood sugar. Just 1 cup cooked yields about 11 grams of fiber and 15 grams of protein. They are an excellent source of iron, magnesium, and folate.

Cannellini beans can be bought canned or dried. Dried beans should be stored in an airtight container and have a very long shelf life. Cannellini beans should be rinsed and then soaked overnight before cooking. You can boil, slow-cook, or pressure-cook these beans. One cup of dried cannellini beans will yield approximately three cups of cooked beans. In recipes that call for this white bean, you can substitute great northern or navy beans. After cooking the beans, they can be added to soups, stews, and chilis or just served with your favorite seasonings. They can even be puréed to a paste and seasoned to serve on crackers or sandwiches.

Nuts for Desserts

The people of the Mediterranean are not big on sweets. Though they may indulge a little, nuts are one of their star dessert ingredients. Traditional Mediterranean cuisine relies heavily on its use of unprocessed foods such as nuts, making their desserts dramatically different than the cookies, cakes, pies, and other high-fat and high-sugar desserts so popular in our Western culture. Have no fear, though! There is just something about that nutty crunch while eating delicious desserts that will still satisfy and delight you and, better yet, fulfill your dietary requirements without leaving you wanting more when your meal is over. Check out the yummy dessert recipes in Chapter 22.

Tips for Adding More Nuts, Seeds, and Legumes to Your Diet

The Mediterranean diet encourages more nuts, seeds, and legumes as part of your daily diet. These may be foods you haven't thought much about until now, so here are a few helpful hints before you get started. As you add more legumes to your diet, be sure to drink enough water to help your digestive system handle the increase in fiber. Keep in mind that nuts and seeds are high in calories, so eat them in moderation. Try the following tips to ensure that you are adding these healthy foods on a daily basis:

- Add legumes to soups, stews, chilis, and casseroles. Even if your recipe doesn't call for them, try adding some for flavor and a nutritional boost.

- Try puréed beans as the basis for dips or season for spreads on flatbreads. Hummus is an example of a spread that uses puréed beans called garbanzo beans. (See Chapter 17 for a hummus recipe.)

- Add cooked dried beans such as chickpeas, kidney beans, or black beans to salads. You can also toss in nuts or seeds to add a little extra crunch.

- Use canned beans instead of dried beans. They can be just as nutritious and are often more convenient. Drain and rinse the canned beans before using to lower the sodium content.

- Eat a handful of nuts or seeds as a quick snack.

- Sprinkle chopped nuts on top of your favorite yogurt.

- Use crushed nuts as a coating for chicken or fish instead of breadcrumbs.

- Use nuts in pasta or vegetable dishes to add flavor and crunch.

- Top your morning oatmeal or cold cereal with a few walnuts, almonds, or other favorite nut.

- Top your favorite cheese with chopped nuts as an appetizer.

- Add ground nuts to homemade bread or muffins.

The Least You Need to Know

- Nuts, seeds, and legumes are an essential component of the plant-based group on the Mediterranean Diet Pyramid.
- Nuts, seeds, and legumes all contribute to heart health and offer many other health benefits as well.
- Some nuts, seeds, and legumes provide the plant-based omega-3 fatty acids (ALA).
- Legumes are high in protein, fiber, phytonutrients, and other essential nutrients for good health. They are also a good substitute for meat.
- Nuts are a main ingredient in many Mediterranean desserts.
- Adding more nuts, seeds, and legumes to your daily diet is easier than you might think.

The "Other" Proteins

In This Chapter

- Exploring more protein choices
- How meat and poultry fit in
- Selecting the leanest meats
- The versatile egg
- Dishing up the dairy

The Mediterranean diet is chock-full of healthy protein sources. The majority of these protein sources come from seafood, grains, legumes, nuts, and seeds with a smaller portion coming from other sources including meat, poultry, eggs, cheese, yogurt, and milk. These other sources can be a bit scary in that you can most definitely find some very unhealthy food choices within them. The key is learning how to choose foods from each of these groups that are indeed healthier and associated with the Mediterranean diet concept.

Meat and Poultry

Meat and poultry do not play a huge role in the Mediterranean diet, but they do indeed play a part. Meat and poultry are acceptable protein choices on the Mediterranean diet. However, depending on cut, grade, and preparation, meat and poultry can add a lot of saturated fat and cholesterol to your diet—so the right choice means everything. One step up on the Mediterranean Diet Pyramid from seafood is the poultry, eggs, cheese, and yogurt group, and one step up from that is the red meat group at the very top of the pyramid, along with sweets. The higher up on the pyramid you go, the less consumed those foods are (see Chapter 3 for more on the pyramid).

Poultry is recommended in moderate portions, every two days or weekly. It is suggested you bake or broil your poultry, as deep-fried foods don't fit into the Mediterranean diet at all. Red meat, at the top of the pyramid, is recommended less often—preferably no more than a few times per month. Specifically, consumption should be limited to a maximum of 12 to 16 ounces per month with leaner versions being the preferred choice. Red meat contains a lot of saturated fat and cholesterol, both of which are bad for your heart and not fitting on a heart-healthy diet. However, there are plenty of healthy protein choices that are heart healthy and that make perfect substitutions. If you must have a burger, try making it out of ground turkey or chicken breast instead of ground beef to cut out a ton of saturated fat and cholesterol.

When it comes to moderation of portion size, forget your 12-ounce steak. To visualize a reasonable portion of meat, three ounces is about the size of the palm of your hand or a deck of playing cards. Try including smaller portions of meat with meals, and for this diet, think of meat as more of a side dish with vegetables and whole grains taking up the majority of your plate.

HEALTHY MORSELS

Here are the government guidelines for meats per $3\frac{1}{2}$ ounce serving:

- **Lean:** Less than 10 grams of total fat, less than 4.5 grams saturated fat, and less than 95 mg of cholesterol.
- **Extra lean:** Less than 5 grams of total fat, less than 2 grams of saturated fat, and less than 95 mg of cholesterol.

Nutritional Properties of Meat

Meat may have its good and bad points, but on the good side, it does provide essential nutrients that are vital for health and maintenance of our bodies. On the bad side, choosing the wrong foods from this group can provide saturated fat and cholesterol, both of which have health implications. Meat and poultry provide a long list of nutrients including B vitamins (niacin, thiamin, riboflavin, and B_6), vitamin E, zinc, and magnesium. Poultry contains a generous portion of some B vitamins that might not be as plentiful in red meat, but it does not contain as much iron as red meat.

Meat can provide a large proportion of our daily protein requirements. Animal protein is known as a complete protein, meaning it contains an ample amount of all the essential amino acids (building blocks of protein) that our body needs to function properly on a daily basis. There are 20 different amino acids, and 9 of these are essential because our bodies cannot make them; therefore, we must get them from the foods we eat. Incomplete proteins (grains, legumes, nuts, seeds, and vegetables) are missing a few essential amino acids or do not have enough of these amino acids. You can still get all of the essential amino acids you need without eating animal protein by eating a large variety of plant foods. If you don't eat meat, you can still get complete proteins in eggs, milk, cheese, seafood, soy, and a few select grains such as quinoa (although grains have a lower Protein Digestibility Corrected Amino Acid Score [PDCAAS], making them a lower-quality protein than some of the others listed). Red meat, in particular, is a large contributor of iron in our diets. Other meats do contain iron, but red meat contains the most. Iron is used in the body to carry oxygen to organs, tissue, and blood. People who do not get enough iron, especially teenage girls and women in their child-bearing years, may suffer from iron-deficiency anemia. Anemia can cause weakness, fatigue, a weakened immune system, and a general feeling of illness. This population should eat foods high in *heme iron*, such as meat, poultry, and fish; or eat foods with *nonheme iron*, such as fruits, vegetables, grains, and nuts, along with foods rich in vitamin C, which can help absorption of the iron.

DEFINITION

Heme iron is the form of most iron found in animal foods and is much more absorbable than the iron found in plant foods (known as **nonheme iron**). Eating an abundance of iron-rich plant foods can ensure that you will meet your daily requirement, but eating meat enhances the absorption of nonheme iron from plant foods.

Common Meats of the Mediterranean

The Mediterranean diet may not revolve around meat, but it does have a place for it. People of the Mediterranean do eat small amounts of meat and even smaller amounts of red meat. The meat that shows up in the traditional diet includes chicken, turkey, duck, guinea fowl, pork, lean beef, lamb, veal, and even mutton and goat—although these are not popular in the American diet.

Duck can be considered a lean poultry if you stick to the breast meat, remove all skin, and drain any fat. Guinea fowl makes a great alternative to chicken and can be cooked in any way that a small chicken would be cooked, such as roasting. This meat has a subtle gamy flavor and is high in protein and low in cholesterol. Lamb is nutrient-dense and lean with very little marbling or fat; however, it contains some monounsaturated and polyunsaturated fats, which are very beneficial.

When it comes to meat, the key to the Mediterranean diet is to replace more of your meat and other animal choices with plant protein sources such as beans, nuts, seeds, and grains as well as with seafood. However, this doesn't mean that the Mediterranean diet is a vegetarian diet, and it doesn't mean that you need to replace all of the meat in your diet with plant sources and fish. As long as you ensure that the red meat and poultry choices that you make are lean, you can enjoy meat in moderation along with other sources of protein and can continue to follow the concepts and reap the benefits of the Mediterranean diet.

Best Cuts and Grades to Choose

The solution to including meat in your Mediterranean diet is to make the best choices. To do that you need to know a little more about meats and how to make better choices. To start out, certain meats in the United States, including beef, veal, and lamb, are graded by the USDA according to their marbled fat content (fat that cannot be trimmed away), texture, appearance, and age of the animal. Pork is not graded; however, it is inspected by the USDA Food Safety and Inspection Service (along with all meat, poultry, and eggs). Check the label to find the grade, which will help you to determine fat content. Nutritionally speaking, the nutrient content including vitamins and minerals is the same regardless of the meat's grade.

TO YOUR HEALTH

There are three grades of meat. *Prime* has the most marbled fat and, unfortunately, because of that is usually the most tender and juicy. *Choice* has a moderate fat content, and *Select* has the least amount of marbled fat. For veal and lamb, the grade *Good* is used instead of *Select*.

Poultry such as chicken and turkey offer high-quality protein and can be one of your leanest animal proteins. Other poultry may include duck, pheasant, and quail, which are leaner choices, especially without the skin. Poultry is not always a guaranteed lower-fat alternative to red meat; dark meat with the skin left on can carry tons of fat. For your leanest pick, you need to lose the skin (pure fat) and choose the white meat portions. The breast contains the lowest amount of fat. Trimming excess fat from poultry will also help to cut the fat.

Shopping and Cooking Tips

Although meat contributes some very important nutrients to the diet, it unfortunately has a few downsides, including saturated fats and cholesterol, which can have some serious health implications. Diets high in saturated fats and cholesterol can raise LDL cholesterol or "bad" cholesterol in the blood, raising your risk for cardiovascular disease and stroke. The good news is that by choosing leaner cuts of meat (which are by definition lower in fat, saturated fat, and calories), limiting the amount you eat, and using the correct cooking techniques, you can enjoy meat as part of your regular diet. Consider these tips when shopping for or cooking meat and poultry to ensure the leanest product:

- When buying meats such as beef, pork, lamb, and veal, look for lean and well-trimmed cuts with $\frac{1}{8}$-inch fat trim or less. Lean cuts of beef include top sirloin, top and bottom round roasts, flank steak, or tenderloin; lean cuts of pork include tenderloin, top loin roast, loin rib chops, or center loin chops; lean cuts of lamb include leg, loin chop, arm chop, or foreshanks; lean cuts of veal include rib or loin chop, roast, cutlet, or blade or arm steak.

- Look for the key words *round* or *loin* when shopping for beef and *loin* or *leg* when buying pork or lamb.

- Choose *select* and *choice* cut meats, or look for labels that state *lean* or *extra lean*.

- Both chicken and turkey can be bought ground, but make sure you are buying ground *breast* meat. If it doesn't say *breast*, then it is ground with dark meat and skin and can be just as high in fat as regular ground beef. Other lean cuts of poultry include skinless chicken breast, skinless turkey breast, or skinless Cornish game hen.

- Choose ground beef that is 90 percent lean or higher. Ground round is the leanest, followed by ground sirloin, chuck, and then regular ground beef.

- Be sure you are buying fresh meats. Beef is usually a bright red color. Note the date on the package as well and only buy meat that will still be fresh when you are ready to use it, unless you plan to freeze it immediately for later use.

- Use moist methods of cooking to keep leaner meats from drying out such as braising, stewing, boiling, sautéing, or stir-frying and drain off any fat.

- If using a dry method of cooking, such as baking or grilling, try marinades to tenderize meat and keep it moist while cooking. Choose healthier marinades such as mixtures of herbs, spices, wine, lemon juice, or olive oil.

- Cooking meats will melt away the marbled fat that you are not able to trim away. When cooking meat or poultry in the oven, put it on a rack in a pan so that the fat drips away from the meat.

- After browning ground meat, drain the fat and rinse the ground meat with hot water. Blot with a paper towel to remove even more fat (as well as the water).

- Don't batter meat or poultry or slather them with creamy sauces, which will add fat and calories.

GOOD TO KNOW

Always be careful handling raw meat, cook it thoroughly (especially pork and poultry), and never thaw at room temperature. Wash your hands thoroughly both before and after handling raw meats. Use designated cutting boards for raw meats and wash them, as well as any utensils used to cut the raw meat, thoroughly after each use.

Eggs

Eggs are another high-quality protein source that is used on the Mediterranean diet. Eggs are grouped with poultry, cheese, and yogurt on the Mediterranean Diet Pyramid with it stating that poultry and eggs be consumed in moderate portions every two days or weekly. The pyramid specifically recommends consuming up to seven eggs per week, including those used in cooking and baking. With their high protein content, eggs are included in the meat, fish, poultry, nuts, and beans group of the USDA's MyPyramid.

Nutritional Properties of Eggs

Eggs are an inexpensive, convenient, and easy-to-prepare source of protein. A large egg provides about 6 grams of high-quality or complete protein. In fact, eggs contain one of the highest-quality proteins. Eggs are very nutrient-dense and low in calories, supplying only about 70 calories for one large egg. Besides protein they are a good source of folate; riboflavin; phosphorus; iron; and vitamins A, D, and B_{12}. Eggs are an excellent source of choline, a vitaminlike substance essential for the normal functioning of all our body's cells. Eggs provide phytonutrients including lutein and zeaxanthin, both of which are included in the carotenoids group. These phytonutrients have been shown to be associated with eye health, skin health, cancer prevention, and slowing the effects of aging. Many of these wonderful nutrients are found in the egg's yolk. The yolk also includes healthy monounsaturated and poly-unsaturated fats; about half of the egg's total of high-quality protein is found there as well.

Because eggs are high in cholesterol—about 213 mg per egg yolk—the American Heart Association recommends monitoring the use of them and limiting cholesterol intake to no more than 300 mg per day. However, the cholesterol in eggs shouldn't scare you away from eating them. If you stick with the recommendations of the Mediterranean diet of no more than seven eggs per week, and you follow the remainder of the diet (which is quite low in cholesterol), eggs can fit in just fine—and you won't be missing out on all the beneficial nutrients they provide.

> **TO YOUR HEALTH**
>
> You can reduce some of the fat and cholesterol in eggs by using one whole egg and extra egg whites when preparing eggs. All of the cholesterol and most of the fat is contained in the yolk of the egg.

Eggs of the Mediterranean

When we think of eggs, we think mostly of eggs from the chicken. In the Mediterranean, they often come from quail and duck as well. Quail eggs are much smaller than chicken eggs and are touted as being among the most delicious. Duck and quail eggs are hard to come by in the United States, but they may be found in specialty food stores.

Eggs have a stronger presence in the traditional Mediterranean diet than meat does. They are used for omelets, sauces, soups, dessert recipes, and for cooking and baking in general. In addition they are used boiled for stuffing in tomatoes or as a breakfast food with chopped tomatoes and other veggies.

Dairy Products

Dairy products are consumed in low to moderate amounts on the Mediterranean diet, with cheese and yogurt being grouped with poultry and eggs on the Mediterranean Diet Pyramid. Dairy foods such as cheese, yogurt, and milk are good sources of calcium, but they can be high in saturated fats because they are animal foods.

Though consumed daily, dairy is not a big part of the traditional Mediterranean diet compared to the typical American diet. People of the Mediterranean get some calcium from dairy but also from alternative plant-based sources such as dark green leafy vegetables, figs, seeds, almonds, tofu, and various beans.

The Mediterranean Diet Pyramid specifies daily consumption of cheese and yogurt (low-fat and fat-free versions are preferable) in low to moderate portions. More specifically, two servings (or more depending on your individual needs) are recommended per day, with a serving equaling one cup of low-fat or fat-free milk, one cup of low-fat or fat-free yogurt, or one ounce of low-fat cheese.

HEALTHY MORSELS

The Dietary Guidelines for Americans and MyPyramid recognize the importance of dairy products as well and recommend three servings a day of milk, cheese, or yogurt in low-fat and fat-free versions.

Nutritional Properties of Dairy Foods

Dairy products are one of the biggest sources of calcium, but that isn't all they provide. Dairy foods are a good source of potassium; phosphorus; protein; riboflavin; niacin; and vitamins A, D, and B_{12}. Beyond containing calcium, which helps to strengthen bones and decreases your risk for osteoporosis, nutrient-rich dairy products can help improve overall nutrient intake and help reduce the risk for chronic health problems such as hypertension. In addition, getting enough dairy may play a role in helping to maintain a healthy weight.

It's not only the amount of protein in dairy but also the source of its protein that is important. Not all proteins are created equal. The proteins in milk, casein, and whey are high quality—meaning they are complete proteins. Adequate intake of high-quality protein, especially whey protein, combined with resistance exercise has been shown to increase muscle mass and promote fat loss. Another good reason to get your dairy in!

Cheese

When we are talking about cheese on the Mediterranean diet, it is not the processed slices that are individually wrapped but rather flavorful and natural cheeses. Cheese in the Mediterranean commonly comes from sheep's and goat's milk, which are usually lower in cholesterol than those made from cow's milk. Since cheese is made from milk, it is a great source of milk's natural nutrients including calcium and protein.

Cheeses common to the Mediterranean include Brie, chèvre, Corvo, feta, fontina, goat, manchego, mozzarella, Parmesan, Parmigiano-Reggiano, ricotta, and pecorino, just to name a few. The cheese you choose should not be processed cheese and it should be naturally low in fat or a lower-fat version, if possible, to cut back on saturated fat. Some of the cheeses common to the Mediterranean may not be low in fat but because many are so flavorful you actually don't need to use too much of it.

TO YOUR HEALTH

When it comes to cheese labeling, *low-fat cheese* has 3 grams of fat or less per serving; *reduced-fat cheese* has 25 percent less fat than the same full-fat cheese; and *fat-free cheese* has less than 0.5 grams of fat per serving.

Yogurt

Yogurt is a nutritious food that, besides protein, calcium, and its other essential nutrients, contains "friendly" or "good" live bacterial cultures that may contribute to good health. These live active cultures may boost the immune system and aid in digestion. Be sure the label states "Live and Active Cultures" before purchasing yogurt.

Yogurt is quite popular in the Mediterranean regions; however, it's not the fruited yogurt we might find at our local grocery store but basic plain yogurt or Greek yogurt. Greek yogurt is much thicker and creamier than the yogurt we are used to eating. In Greece, this yogurt is usually made from sheep's or cow's milk, but most of the Greek yogurt in the United States is made from cow's milk. Making Greek yogurt requires a few extra steps, with one of the important ones being a filtering or straining process, which gives the yogurt a thicker consistency. Greek yogurt tends to be a bit higher in protein and lower in sugar. However, just as with regular yogurt, stay away from the full fat versions, which can be high in saturated fats.

In the Mediterranean, yogurt is used for more than just breakfast or a quick snack. It is quite popular in the Mediterranean regions to sweeten yogurt naturally with fresh fruit or honey. Plain yogurt or Greek yogurt are used in dips, sauces, and dressings and are served with meat and vegetables. A popular Greek dip called tzatziki is made with yogurt and is used as a dip, spread, or condiment (see Chapter 19 for a recipe that features tzatziki).

Milk

Milk certainly plays a role in a healthy diet, but for those in the Mediterranean regions, it usually is not the beverage of choice. In the Mediterranean, milk is used more frequently in preparing foods than for drinking. Most dairy foods are consumed in the form of cheese or yogurt. However, if you are a milk drinker, then using low-fat or fat-free milk can definitely be a part of a healthy Mediterranean diet as long as guidelines are followed.

The Least You Need to Know

- Meat and poultry are consumed on the Mediterranean diet as a protein source but in moderation and not on a daily basis.
- The leanest cuts of meat and poultry should be used when including them on the Mediterranean diet. Poultry is favored over red meat, which is placed at the very top of the Mediterranean Diet Pyramid.
- Consumed in moderation, eggs contribute high-quality protein as well as a host of other essential nutrients and can be part of this healthy diet.
- Cheese is a common dairy choice, with most cheese coming from sheep's or goat's milk. Processed cheese is not part of this diet.
- Both Greek and plain yogurts (in low-fat versions) are common dairy choices. Milk is not the beverage of choice but is used quite often in preparing meals.

Add Spice to Your Life

In This Chapter

- Spark up your meals the Mediterranean way
- Herbs and spices used in Mediterranean cooking
- The heart-healthy benefits of wine
- Wine and the Mediterranean diet
- Nonalcoholic alternatives

The Mediterranean diet is all about flavor. Not only is it the foods that add to this diet, but also the large array of flavorful herbs and spices that are so commonly used. A pinch of this and a dash of that adds flavor to your favorite dishes and gives them a Mediterranean flair while adding a host of health benefits. It's hard to say who invented wine, but we do know that societies have enjoyed this beverage throughout history. On the Mediterranean diet, wine is more than just a stress reliever after a long day at work—it's a beneficial and key component to the diet's healthy benefits. Wine has traditionally been consumed by people living in the countries bordering the Mediterranean Sea for centuries, and their good health points to the potential benefits of drinking moderate amounts of red wine. (If you're not a wine drinker, you'll be happy to know that drinking purple grape juice offers many of the same healthy benefits.)

Spice Up Your Foods!

Herbs and spices are used liberally in Mediterranean cooking and have been a culinary tradition in these areas for thousands of years. In fact, they are so essential to the Mediterranean diet that the new Mediterranean Diet Pyramid has added herbs and spices to its dietary guidelines. New evidence-based research has proven that they may just possess health-promoting characteristics. These tasty additions to your favorite recipes are rich in a broad range of antioxidants and phytonutrients. Herbs and spices add plenty in the way of flavor and aroma to foods (not to mention helping to retain flavor in foods) while reducing the need for salt, fat, and sugar.

Although the terms *herb* and *spice* are often used interchangeably, they are not the same. By definition, herbs are the fragrant leaves of plants or low-growing shrubs. Examples include thyme, basil, dill, oregano, and rosemary. Herbs can be used fresh or dried, with dried forms being either whole, crushed, or ground. Spices, on the other hand, come from the bark, root, buds, seeds, stems, berries, or fruit of plants or trees. They normally come in only a dried version (except for garlic and ginger root, which come in other varieties such as cloves). Other examples of spices are paprika, allspice, and coriander. Seasoning blends are usually a mixture of both herbs and spices.

GOOD TO KNOW

Some seasonings can contain quite a bit of sodium, such as garlic salt, celery salt, onion salt, or seasoned salt. Use these sparingly and be sure to read the food label.

Herbs and Spices Common to the Mediterranean

There are many herbs and spices common to the Mediterranean, but keep in mind that whether they are common to the Mediterranean or not, they can be a healthy part of your diet. Try your favorite or experiment with something new. Either way, herbs and spices can add plenty of flavor, originality, and appeal to your foods and meals—and a boost of nutrition as well!

Popular herbs and spices of the Mediterranean include anise, basil, bay leaf, cardamom, cilantro, chilies, clove, cumin, dill, fennel, fenugreek, garlic, ginger, lavender, marjoram, mint, oregano, paprika, parsley, pepper, red pepper flakes, rosemary, saffron, sage, savory, sumac, tarragon, turmeric, thyme, and zatar.

Here are some ideas for spicing up snacks and meals with Mediterranean flavor:

- Add rosemary to roasted potatoes for a great side dish for meats or fish.

- Add crushed red pepper, paprika, or fresh garlic to hummus.

- Roll a log of goat cheese in cracked black pepper, chili powder, oregano, basil, thyme, or dill. Serve as an appetizer with olives, dried fruit, nuts, or grapes.

- Top fresh tomatoes with balsamic vinegar and extra-virgin olive oil. Add fresh chopped garlic and a dash of fresh or dried basil or oregano. Toss and serve along fish or meat or on top of salad greens.

- Add finely chopped fresh mint to your favorite mix of fresh fruit.

- Add oregano to whole-wheat pasta and drizzle with olive oil. Add your favorite veggies.

- Top your favorite rolls with olive oil, rosemary, and sea salt.

- Add a pinch of thyme to your eggs before cooking.

- Add a sprinkle of thyme to lamb or pork chops before grilling.

- Sauté steamed spinach, garlic, and fresh lemon juice for a tasty side dish.

The possibilities are endless when it comes to adding herbs and spices to your recipes and foods. Experiment by adding them slowly and using a variety of mixtures—and boost your antioxidant intake at the same time.

Fresh herbs can be wonderful in cooking; however, sometimes they can be hard to find or expensive unless you grow your own. Dried is a great alternative, but because dried herbs are much stronger than fresh versions, different amounts should be used when cooking. As a general rule of thumb, you can substitute one teaspoon of dried herbs for one tablespoon of fresh herbs and vice versa. Let your personal taste be your guide!

GOOD TO KNOW

A few simple herbs and spices can help bring out the flavor of foods, but adding too much can overwhelm your dish. If you're not sure about flavor or strength, start with just ¼ teaspoon of dried herbs or spices per 1 pound of meat. You can always add more—but once you add it, you can't take it away!

Dried herbs and spices can spoil within a year. Buy only what you will use within a few months; check the date on the container; store in a tightly covered container; store in a cool, dark, dry place; and do not refrigerate.

The following sections look at a few of the most common herbs and spices used in Mediterranean cooking. You may already use some of these, but you may find a few new ideas.

Garlic

Garlic is a versatile seasoning and a customary addition in Mediterranean cuisine in sauces, stews, soups, cooked vegetables, salad dressings, casseroles, and grain dishes. It is also used on bread and for marinades or rubs. Garlic can come fresh (cloves), dried, minced, or in powder form. Numerous studies have found that regular consumption of garlic can potentially help to decrease cholesterol and triglyceride levels, therefore lowering the risk for heart disease. Studies show that it may even help to lower blood pressure and prevent certain types of cancer. Garlic gets its potential health benefits from sulfur compounds called *allicin* and *diallyl disulphide.* Allicin is what gives garlic its pungent odor. This compound is a powerful antibacterial and antiviral agent that has been shown to protect against common infections like colds, flu, and some stomach viruses. Diallyl disulphide is also responsible for that strong garlic odor. This compound offers an antimicrobial effect as well as protection against colon cancer and cardiovascular disease. Other helpful nutrients are vitamin C and selenium, both of which are antioxidants; and manganese and vitamin B_6.

Mint

Mint is known to have originated in the Mediterranean regions, with spearmint and peppermint being the most widely used varieties. It is highly fragrant and best used fresh, though dried is also available. Mint is full of essential vitamins, antioxidants, and minerals including vitamin A (beta-carotene), vitamin C, thiamin, folate, riboflavin, manganese, magnesium, copper, potassium, iron, calcium, zinc, and phosphorus. With its rich nutritional content, it has many health benefits. Mint has been used for centuries to aid in digestion and to help relieve indigestion. In addition, it may help protect against certain cancers, inhibit the growth of bacteria and fungus, combat bad breath, relieve congestion, and ease breathing.

Both peppermint and spearmint are quite widely used in Mediterranean cuisine and add a fresh flavor to a variety of sweet and savory dishes. Mint, especially spearmint, is added to eggs, hot and cold teas, sauces, dressings (especially yogurt dressings), salads, cooked vegetables, stews, soups, stuffings, and fruits. Mint can be used in marinades for lamb or fish and added to rice, couscous, or bean dishes. A popular salad dish, tabbouleh, contains mint. Because of peppermint's strong aroma and flavor, it is popular mostly in dessert dishes.

Thyme

Thyme is native to and widely used in Mediterranean cuisine. It has a highly aromatic scent, so it should be used sparingly. It can be used both fresh and dried. Thyme adds not only a burst of flavor to foods, it is also filled with nutrients including phytonutrients and flavonoids. These nutrients act as powerful antioxidants, which means they protect against free radicals and help to protect the cells of our bodies from chronic disease such as heart disease and cancer. This herb also contains iron; manganese; calcium; some dietary fiber; and vitamins A, C, and K. Thyme may benefit respiratory problems and aid in digestion. It also has antibacterial and antifungal properties. Thyme is popularly used with tomato-based dishes and in soups, sauces, stuffings, and marinades. It makes a great addition to egg, bean, and vegetable dishes, and also pairs well with poultry, seafood, and meats.

For longer staying power, treat fresh herbs like fresh flowers. Chop off the bottom edges of the stems, just like you would with fresh flowers. Place in a glass filled with water to just cover the stems. You can leave them out on the counter or place them in the refrigerator door if your kitchen is warm. They'll last up to a week.

Why Is Wine Heart Healthy?

The benefits of red wine have often been studied. Researchers have discovered that even though the French eat a diet high in saturated fats—with butter, croissants, creamy sauces, cheese, and other fatty delights—statistically they have a significantly lower incidence of deaths from heart disease. Researchers have concluded that the mitigating factor in all of this was the French people's regular consumption of wine.

It isn't just wine in general but red wine specifically that studies are now suggesting protect against heart disease. Studies suggest that drinking red wine may have blood-thinning and anticlotting properties that help to lower the risk of heart attack and stroke in middle-age people. It may also help prevent additional heart attacks after already suffering from one. Other studies have indicated that red wine can help raise HDL (or good cholesterol) in the blood stream, which acts as a protector for the heart and can help prevent artery damage by lowering blood levels of LDL (or bad cholesterol)—it may even prevent LDL from forming.

A growing body of scientific research shows that wine is not just good for your heart but also offers health protection in other ways as well. The phytonutrients found in red wine offer a significant boost of antioxidant protection, which has the potential to help prevent not only heart disease but also various forms of cancer (such as colon cancer) by inhibiting tumor development. Other studies have found that these phyto-nutrients may be helpful in the treatment of neurological diseases such as Parkinson's and Alzheimer's diseases and age-related memory loss. Research continues on the health links to red wine, but so far things are looking positive.

> **TO YOUR HEALTH**
>
> Wine is not the cure-all. The health benefits of drinking moderate amounts of wine are enhanced when you eat a heart-healthy diet, exercise regularly, and eliminate harmful lifestyle habits such as smoking.

Nutritional Properties of Wine

It's no wonder that wine provides some health benefits—it comes from the grape, a fruit that is loaded with vitamins, minerals, antioxidants, and phytonutrients. Wine, especially red wine, contains loads of health-promoting phytonutrients. Two of the most powerful in red wine are subclasses of polyphenols, including resveratrol and flavonoids. Other foods rich in polyphenols include onions, apples, green tea, broccoli, red peppers, red grapes, red grape juice, strawberries, blueberries, cranberries, some nuts, and even olive oil (especially extra-virgin olive oil). Experts believe that polyphenols may help to prevent chronic diseases such as cancer, heart disease, and inflammation.

Other phytonutrients called saponins have also been found to be more concentrated in red wine. This compound is believed to prevent the absorption of cholesterol into the blood stream and to act as an anti-inflammatory, having implications in not only heart disease but cancer as well. Saponins can also be found in olive oil and soybeans. Proanthocyanidins can be found in red wine as well as in grapes, grape juice, tea, cocoa, many berries, and cranberries and cranberry juice. This phytonutrient may also help reduce the risk of heart disease and cancer as well as protect against urinary tract infections.

Tannins are also associated with wine and found in the skins, seeds, and stems of grapes. Because the skins supply color to the wine, red wines typically contain more tannin than white wines. Tannins act as a natural preservative for wine and give wine structure and texture. Tannins offer heart-healthy benefits and may also inhibit plate-let clotting. Tannins can also be found in tea, coffee beans, certain fruits, chocolate, and some nuts.

GOOD TO KNOW

Red wine can trigger migraine headaches in people who are susceptible or sensitive to it, and some experts believe tannins are responsible. French red wines (especially Bordeaux), Italian reds (especially Barolo and Barbaresco), and wines made from cabernet sauvignon grapes are high in tannins. Wines lower in tannins include Burgundy and dolcetto, and wines made from pinot noir, Barbera, and Sangiovese grapes.

Flavonoids

Flavonoids are a subclass of polyphenols, which are among the most potent and abundant in our food supply. More than 4,000 types of flavonoids have been identified. The flavonoids are further divided into subclasses depending on their differences in chemical structure. Catechin is an important flavonoid that is related to the subgroup called flavanols. It's abundant in red wine and is found to reduce the risk of heart disease by exhibiting significant antioxidant power that may help prevent blood clots and the formation of plaque in the arteries. It also seems to play a role in healthy lung function. Catechins can also be found in green, black, and white tea; cocoa powder; dark chocolate; grapes; and plums.

Resveratrol

Resveratrol falls under the nonflavonoid subclass of polyphenols. It is believed that resveratrol is one of the compounds responsible for the health benefits associated with the Mediterranean diet. It seems to be the key ingredient in red wine that helps to prevent damage to blood vessels, reduce inflammation, increase HDL cholesterol, reduce LDL cholesterol, and prevent blood clots. In addition, resveratrol has been demonstrated to be a potent antioxidant and have anticancer effects as well. If you are not a wine drinker, you can also find resveratrol in grape skin and juice, peanuts, blueberries, and cranberries.

How Wine Figures into the Mediterranean Diet

Wine is a popular beverage throughout the Mediterranean and is a staple of the diet there. Throughout the years, studies have shown that people from the Mediterranean regions who regularly consume red wine have lower risks of heart disease. Although it is consumed regularly, it is consumed in moderation. The guidelines of the Mediterranean Diet Pyramid suggest moderate consumption of wine, normally with meals, amounting to about one to two glasses per day for men and one glass per day for women (one glass equals five ounces). The pyramid also states that, from a contemporary public health perspective, wine should be considered optional and avoided when consumption puts an individual or others at risk. Wine is enjoyed with meals in the Mediterranean; recreational drinking is typically not part of the Mediterranean lifestyle.

GOOD TO KNOW

If you have problems limiting your alcohol intake to the amounts recommended for good health, are pregnant, have a personal or family history of alcohol abuse, have heart or liver disease, have any other medical or health condition that warrants not drinking alcohol, or are on certain prescription medications, refrain from drinking wine or any other type of alcohol. If you have concerns, speak with your health-care provider.

Which Wines Are Best for Heart Health?

Many of the heart-healthy phytonutrients found in wine, including resveratrol and other polyphenols, are present in the skin and seeds of the grape. Because the skin is used in fermentation of red wine, the amount of health-promoting phytonutrients is much higher than in white or rosé wines, where the grape skins are removed earlier in the process. In rosé wines, the skin is left on just a bit longer than with white wines. This gives them that rosy color and allows them to offer a bit more in the way of health benefits than white wine, but not nearly as much as red wine. The longer the grape skin is used in the fermentation process, the more phytonutrients the wine will contain.

Though red wine is a good source of phytonutrients, not all red wines contain the same amount. The amount of these phytonutrients (such as resveratrol) is not measured frequently in most wines, and it can change from year to year depending on growing conditions of the grapes. Additionally, the phytonutrient levels in wine can deteriorate over time, so drinking younger wines may be more beneficial.

Several studies say cabernet sauvignon and pinot noir seem to be the highest in phytonutrients. If you are not a red wine drinker, switching from white wine might take some getting used to. In this case, you might go for a lighter red such as merlot.

Choose red wines that are darker and have a more intense color and flavor as this will generally indicate higher levels of phytonutrients. When possible, favor wines straight from the Mediterranean regions, particularly from southern France, Greece, Sardinia, Sicily, and other places in the southern part of Italy.

Classifications of Red Wine

Red wines are classified as light-bodied, medium-bodied, or full-bodied. The *bodied* part of the classification depicts the texture of the wine, while the light, medium, and full describes the weight that you might feel on your tongue when you drink the wine.

- **Light-bodied wines** have fewer tannins and so have a milder flavor and mouthfeel. These wines tend to go better with boldly flavored foods and are typically lower in alcohol content. Examples of light-bodied wines include beaujolais nouveau, pinot noir, and red burgundy.

- **Medium-bodied wines** contain more tannins and so will be in the middle of the road when it comes to robust flavor, texture, and mouthfeel. Examples of medium-bodied wines include merlot, shiraz, and chianti.

- **Full-bodied wines** boast the highest tannin and alcohol content and so will give you stronger flavor with a heavier mouthfeel. Examples of full-bodied wines include bordeaux, cabernet sauvignon, and zinfandel.

TO YOUR HEALTH

Most red wines taste best when served at about 65°F, which is a bit cooler than room temperature. They are best stored in a cellar or basement; if not, they should be chilled shortly before serving.

What About White Wines?

Although white wine doesn't boast the health-promoting phytonutrient content that red wine does, most alcohol in moderation does have some benefits. White wines are usually a yellow or golden color and are made from an assortment of grape varietals. White wines are made from the juice and skin of green, gold, or yellow-colored grapes. They can also be made from the juice, but not the skin, of certain red grapes.

However, because the red color of the skin is where most of the phytonutrients come from, the difference in health benefits between white and red wines is quite substantial. So although your best bet is red wine, moderate alcohol consumption may provide some health benefits such as reducing the risk for heart disease or stroke.

Most white wines are much lighter and have less body than red wines, largely because they lack the tannins of red wines. Some popular white wines include Riesling, sauvignon blanc, pinot grigio, gewurztraminer, and chardonnay. As a rule of thumb, white wines usually go best with lighter meals and foods that have a milder flavor.

Pairing Red Wine with Foods

The people of the Mediterranean enjoy red wine on a regular basis, but it is almost always consumed with meals. There are plenty of red wines to choose from, and you can always find one to go with just about anything you are eating. The key is to take into account what the key ingredients of your entrée will be. Choose a wine that will not distract from or compete with the food you are eating. Wine should add to your meal. There isn't much science behind selection of wine; it is mostly personal preference.

Not quite sure where to start? Here are a few suggestions for some of the more popular red wines. Take these suggestions for what they're worth and don't be afraid to experiment and bend the rules to account for your own preferences. All that matters is that the combination tastes good to you. If you are throwing a dinner party, it is usually best to stick with common pairings so that you know for sure you have a combination that truly works for the majority of people. One quick rule of thumb is to balance flavor intensity. Do this by pairing light-bodied wines with lighter foods and medium- to full-bodied wines with heartier, more flavorful, and richer dishes. A wonderful pairing with wine is cheese. Hard cheeses are usually stronger in flavor and tend to go better with red wines. Softer cheese, usually milder in flavor, pairs better with white wines.

- **Cabernet sauvignon** is best with beef or steak, duck, roasts, spicy poultry, lamb, lentils, or strongly flavored cheeses such as cheddar or blue cheese.

- **Merlot** is best with veal, lamb, stew, salmon, tuna, beef, strong or aged cheese, pastas with red sauces, heavy seafoods, barbequed chicken, or pork.

- **Zinfandel** is best with duck, beef, tomato sauce, or barbeque sauce.

- **Pinot noir** is best with veal, chicken, turkey, lean cuts of beef, lamb, salmon, or tuna.

- **Syrah/Shiraz** is best with lamb, meat stew, pasta with tomato sauce, barbeque sauces, and spicy dishes.

- **Chianti** is best with Italian dishes, tomato-based sauces, poultry, and steak.

Everything in Moderation

It is important to reiterate that the guidelines of the Mediterranean Diet Pyramid suggest moderate consumption of wine, normally with meals, amounting to one to two glasses per day for men and one glass per day for women (one glass equals five ounces). The Dietary Guidelines for Americans advises that those who choose to drink alcoholic beverages should do so sensibly and in moderation. Experts agree that alcohol should be consumed only in moderation.

Drinking too much alcohol can be addictive for some and is associated with other less favorable health issues. Drinking more alcohol than the moderate amount recommended for probable health benefits can increase the risk for high blood pressure, high triglycerides, liver damage, obesity, certain types of cancer, and other problems. In fact, if you have a weakened heart or other major health issues associated with your heart, you should avoid alcohol. If you take aspirin daily, you should avoid or limit your alcohol consumption based on your health-care provider's advice. The benefits discussed in this chapter are associated with consistent, moderate consumption of red wine. Serious health implications are associated with both heavy drinking and sporadic binge drinking. If you are not sure if drinking red wine is right for you, speak with your health-care provider.

 GOOD TO KNOW

The American Heart Association (AHA) cautions people *not* to start drinking if they do not already drink alcohol. If you do drink alcohol, do so in moderation. The AHA recommends an average of one to two drinks per day for men and one drink for women, with five ounces of wine equaling one drink.

What If I Don't Drink?

Red wine's probable health benefits look promising; however, they are certainly no reason to start drinking if you don't already do so. If you don't drink alcohol, there are other ways to get many of the same health benefits of red wine. Several studies have suggested that drinking red or purple grape juice may have some of the same beneficial health effects as drinking red wine. In fact, studies on Concord grapes, which are used to make many brands of grape juice, have been underway for many years and have shown that these grapes are loaded with a vast variety of flavonoids and resveratrol as found in red wine. Grape juice can contain a lot of calories so, just like red wine, drink it in moderation. Also, always read the food label to ensure you are buying 100 percent juice and not a grape drink with added sugar.

Many foods in the purple/blue fruit group have many of the same phytonutrients as red wine, including blueberries, blackberries, strawberries, cranberries, purple or red whole grapes, plums (fresh or dried), and eggplant. The majority of fruits and vegetables offer benefits for heart protection and health, so include a variety of fruits and vegetables to maximize heart health and stay physically active.

The Least You Need to Know

- Herbs and spices are used widely in Mediterranean cuisine and are part of the Mediterranean Diet Pyramid.
- Garlic, mint, and thyme are just a few of the common herbs and spices used in Mediterranean cuisine.
- Research shows that red wine has heart-healthy benefits, anticancer effects, and neurological benefits.
- Red wine is loaded with health-promoting phytonutrients, including flavonoids and resveratrol.
- The guidelines of the Mediterranean Diet Pyramid suggest moderate consumption of wine with meals amounting to about one to two glasses per day for men and one glass per day for women (one glass equals five ounces).
- If you don't drink, don't start. Try drinking 100 percent purple grape juice as an alternative.

Treasures of the Mediterranean Diet

The Mediterranean diet is without a doubt one of the healthiest out there. But what is it that makes this diet so good for you? Of course, it is the foods that are consumed, but it's also the Mediterranean lifestyle as a whole. This part clues you in to what is in those foods so popular to the Mediterranean that makes this way of life so healthy for your heart and your overall well-being. You discover all you ever needed to know about fat, fiber, and other essential nutrients that make this not just a diet, but a change to your way of eating that you'll want to adopt as your permanent way of life.

Making Sense of Fat

In This Chapter

- Why we need fat in our diet
- Healthy fats of the Mediterranean diet
- Good versus bad fat
- Make changes that stick

For decades warnings have swirled around the reality of how much fat we eat. We have been taught that low-fat is the best approach to both losing weight and lowering our risk for heart disease. Although we know that fat is an essential nutrient, the Mediterranean diet has proved to us that it is not just the amount of fat we eat but more importantly the *types* of fat we choose. Fat can be a confusing topic with good fats, bad fats, healthy fats, and unhealthy fats. This chapter helps you make sense of it all and better understand how to make fat work in your diet.

Fats *Do* Matter

Some people can't get enough fat and overeat in this food category; others fear fat and take it to the extreme by eating little or no fat. The key is balance and sticking to a diet made up of mostly healthy fats. Fats do matter in our diet. They are an essential nutrient and we could not survive without them. Here are a few jobs they have in the body:

- Fat, along with carbohydrates and protein, provides the body with a source of energy to power physical activity and basic functions that keep our body going.

- Fat supports cell growth and aids in the production of important hormones.

- Fat enables the fat-soluble vitamins A, D, E, and K and the phytonutrient carotenoids to be transported and absorbed through the bloodstream. Without fat in our diet, we would be deficient in these nutrients.

- Fat supplies essential fatty acids that our bodies cannot make—we must get it from the foods we eat.

- Fat helps to promote healthy skin and hair.

- Fat supports and protects our vital organs and bones from injury and provides insulation as a fat layer under the skin, which keeps us warm on cold days.

- Fat adds flavor and aroma to foods and satiety to our diets.

How the Mediterranean Diet Delivers Healthy Fats

People of the Mediterranean regions certainly eat their fair share of fat, but it comes in the form of healthy fats and is balanced with other healthy foods, moderate portions, and regular physical activity. A low-fat diet may not always be the way to go as these diets can be lacking enough of these healthy fats. Thanks to the Mediterranean diet the word *fat* doesn't seem quite so scary anymore. Even though the Mediterranean diet adds up to about 40 percent of total daily calories from fat sources, those fat sources contain mostly healthy fats.

Olive oil is the primary fat source in Mediterranean foods and cooking. As you learned in Chapter 6, olive oil is full of monounsaturated fats that, when used in place of unhealthy fats, have been proven to be heart healthy. Other healthy fats of the Mediterranean diet include polyunsaturated fats and omega-3 fatty acids, which are found in fish, seafood, nuts, seeds, and other vegetable oils.

How does the Mediterranean diet compare to others when it comes to fat intake?

The American Heart Association recommends:

- Limit fat intake to less than 25 to 35 percent of total daily calories.

- Limit saturated fat intake to less than 7 percent of total daily calories with the rest coming from polyunsaturated and monounsaturated fats such as nuts, seeds, fish, and vegetable oils.

The Dietary Guidelines for Americans recommends:

- Keep total fat intake between 20 to 35 percent of total daily calories with most sources coming from polyunsaturated and monounsaturated fats such as fish, nuts, and vegetable oils.

- Consume less than 10 percent of total daily calories from saturated fat.

The Mediterranean diet is obviously higher in fat, but it is not the amount of fat that is the issue as much as it is the type of fat that is more commonly consumed. The Mediterranean diet is much higher in monounsaturated fats than the typical Western diet, with well over half of the fat calories coming directly from monounsaturated fats. The average American fat intake is about 35 to 40 percent with a good majority coming from saturated fats. The idea is not to simply add healthy fat sources to the foods you already eat but to replace the bad fats in your diet with good fats.

HEALTHY MORSELS

Olive oil, the most commonly used fat in the Mediterranean diet, contains zero trans fat and is lower in saturated fat than many other commonly used fats such as butter or shortening.

What Are Fats?

All fats belong to a group called *lipids*, a general term that refers to all fats, cholesterol, and fatlike substances. In scientific terms, fats are chains of carbon, hydrogen, and oxygen.

Some fats are solid at room temperature while others are liquid. But whether they are solid or liquid, all fat that we consume from food, termed *triglycerides*, is broken down in the body to fatty acids and glycerol. There are three types of fatty acids: saturated, monounsaturated, and polyunsaturated. Most fat-containing foods and oils contain a mixture of these fatty acids and are classified according to the dominant fat. Depending on the proportion of fatty acid content, they will either be liquid (such as olive oil) if they have more unsaturated fats or solid (such as butter) if they have more saturated fats.

GOOD TO KNOW

You may have had your blood triglyceride levels checked by your doctor if you have had a lipid profile or cholesterol test. Besides being found as fat in food, triglycerides also circulate in the bloodstream and are deposited in the body's fat cells. A high triglyceride level can be a risk factor for heart disease.

Not All Fats Are Created Equal

There are many different types of fats, so to make it easier to understand, experts have divided them into just two categories: "good" and "bad." The good guys include monounsaturated fats, polyunsaturated fats, and omega-3 fatty acids. This is the category of fats that is most prevalent in the Mediterranean diet.

Fats are all created equal when it comes to calories. Whether healthy or unhealthy, all fats are higher in calories (9 calories per gram) than carbohydrates and protein (both 4 calories per gram). The biggest difference between fats is that the good fats are healthy fats and have health-promoting effects and the bad fats have the opposite effect.

Monounsaturated Fats

Foods found in the Mediterranean diet are most abundant in monounsaturated fats. Monounsaturated fats are deemed *mono* because they are missing one hydrogen pair on their chemical chain. They are typically liquid at room temperature but will solidify when chilled. These healthy fats are usually a good source of vitamin E, a powerful antioxidant that has been associated with reducing the risk for heart disease. Research shows that monounsaturated fats, when used to replace saturated or trans fats, can help to lower total cholesterol and LDL (bad) blood cholesterol, reducing the risk for heart disease and stroke. Research has also shown that these fats can reduce inflammation and possibly protect from some forms of cancer, as well as help to increase insulin sensitivity, which aids the body in better utilizing glucose or blood sugar.

In addition, because fat takes longer to digest than protein and carbohydrates, these fats can help keep us feeling fuller longer after a meal or snack. Eating too much of the bad fats can pose health problems, but fortunately, unsaturated fats (such as monounsaturated fats) do not pose risks and have health benefits. By adding them to your diet, you will feel fuller and more satisfied, which can help you stick to a healthier diet regimen by making it easier to control portion sizes and eat only at scheduled times.

Foods highest in monounsaturated fatty acids include:

- Olive oil and olives
- Canola and peanut oil
- Sunflower and sesame oil
- Avocados
- Hazelnuts, macadamia nuts, almonds, Brazil nuts, cashews, and pecans
- Sesame seeds and pumpkin seeds
- Peanut butter

Polyunsaturated Fats

Polyunsaturated fats are another healthy fat found in the Mediterranean diet. Polyunsaturated fats are deemed *poly* because, unlike monounsaturated fats, they have more than one missing hydrogen pair on their chemical chain. These fats are typically liquid at room temperature and when chilled. When polyunsaturated fats are consumed in moderation and used to replace saturated fats or trans fats in the diet, they can help reduce total cholesterol, lower LDL (bad) blood cholesterol levels, and lower blood triglyceride levels, thus lowering the risk for heart disease and stroke. These types of unsaturated fats include omega-6 and omega-3 fatty acids, which are essential to our health, but because the body cannot produce them, we must get them from the foods we eat. Polyunsaturated fats have many of the same health benefits as monounsaturated fats.

Foods highest in polyunsaturated fatty acids include:

- Soybean, corn, and safflower oils
- Walnuts, pine nuts, and butternuts
- Sunflower seeds, flaxseeds, and sesame seeds
- Fatty fish and shellfish

Omega-3 Fatty Acids

Omega-3 fatty acids are a group of polyunsaturated fatty acids that provides many health benefits. The Mediterranean diet is loaded with omega-3 fatty acids, which is one of the reasons that people of these regions are so much healthier. These fats play a crucial role in brain function and normal growth and body development. Research shows that omega-3 fatty acids help to reduce inflammation and may have the power to reduce the risk for heart disease, cancer, and arthritis. They may help lower total cholesterol, increase HDL (good) cholesterol, lower triglycerides, lower blood pressure, alleviate some symptoms of depression and other psychological disorders, and improve skin disorders. The list continues to grow as more research is completed.

Omega-3 fatty acids are found mostly in fatty fish such as salmon, mackerel, halibut, tuna, and herring. In fish, they are found in the forms of EPA (eicosapentaeonic acid) and DHA (docoshexaeonic acid), which were both discussed in Chapter 10. These two types of omega-3 fatty acids provide the greatest potential health benefits. Omega-3 fatty acids can also be found in a variety of plant foods, including walnuts, soybeans, flaxseeds, pumpkin seeds, and numerous nut oils. Just two servings a week of foods high in omega-3 fatty acids can give you what you need to reap its health benefits but as with the other healthy fats, they need to not be an addition to your diet but to replace the unhealthier fats. But don't go overboard—too much omega-3, especially in the form of supplements, can have health implications for some people.

TO YOUR HEALTH

New foods on the market today are fortified with omega-3 fatty acids including eggs, yogurt, peanut butter, bread, and pasta. These fortified foods usually contain very little of this healthy fatty acid, and you would need to eat a lot of the food to get the recommended amount. Additional omega-3 fatty acids found in these foods aren't harmful, but you shouldn't substitute these foods for ones that naturally contain omega-3 fatty acids.

Omega-6 Fatty Acids

Omega-6 fatty acids are a group of polyunsaturated fats that you may not have heard much about. They, too, are considered an essential fatty acid because they are necessary for our health; however, our body cannot make them, so we must get them from the foods we eat. Just like omega-3 fatty acids, omega-6 fatty acids play a crucial role in brain function and normal growth and development. When used to replace unhealthy fats, these fatty acids have been shown to also be beneficial in reducing blood cholesterol levels, therefore lowering the risk for heart disease and stroke.

The most common omega-6 fatty acids are linoleic acid (LA) and arachidonic acid (AA). The one we consume the most of, linoleic acid, is found mostly in nuts, seeds, and many vegetable oils, such as soybean, corn, safflower, and sunflower. Because many of these types of refined oils are used in processed foods, they can also be found in many snack foods, cookies, crackers, sweets, and even fast foods. The omega-6 fatty acids we consume the least of can be found in meat, poultry, eggs, and some fish.

There has been much controversy and confusion concerning omega-6 fatty acids. The problem revolves around how much of this fatty acid we should consume, because it is believed that AA has pro-inflammatory properties, which can be linked to heart disease. Some believe these pro-inflammatory properties can be remedied with the proper intake or ratio of omega-3 fatty acids to omega-6 fatty acids.

Experts do agree that omega-6 fatty acids and omega-3 fatty acids should be consumed in varying degrees and that there should be some type of ratio or balance between them. The typical American diet is usually off balance, providing excessive amounts of omega-6 fatty acids and low levels of omega-3 fatty acids. On the contrary, the Mediterranean diet provides a healthier balance between the two fatty acids, making it more heart healthy. The Mediterranean diet is more favorably balanced because it doesn't include as much of the meat, sweets, and processed foods that are high in omega-6 fatty acids. Instead the diet includes more of the foods higher in omega-3 fatty acids and better balances the good foods that do include omega-6 fatty acids.

The key is a proper balance of these omega fatty acids. The solution is not only decreasing the amount of omega-6 fatty acids you consume but also increasing omega-3 fatty acids. In general you can cut back on omega-6 fatty acids and increase omega-3 fatty acids by reducing your consumption of processed foods and fast foods; replacing polyunsaturated vegetable oils with extra-virgin olive oil; and eating less meat and more fish, nuts, and seeds. However, the bottom line is that we do get more LA than AA in most of our diets. Omega-6 fatty acids are essential, are associated with a lower risk for heart disease and stroke, and can be a part of a healthy diet.

The Bad Fats

In the war on fats, the bad guys are saturated fats and trans fats. Fortunately, both of these types of fat are very limited on the Mediterranean diet. Learn a little about each and find out why not having them in your diet can be heart healthy.

Saturated Fats

Saturated fats are most definitely the bad guy. The chemical structure of these fats is fully saturated with hydrogen atoms. This makes saturated fat solid at room temperature, unlike unsaturated fats that are liquid at room temperature. Saturated fats are the main cause of high blood cholesterol levels, even more so than dietary cholesterol. And because many of the foods that are high in saturated fat are also high in cholesterol, it's a double whammy! Saturated fats trigger the liver to make more LDL (bad) cholesterol. This all adds up to a higher risk for heart disease, stroke, and some types of cancer.

Saturated fats are found naturally in most animal-based foods such as meat, poultry, butter, and whole or reduced-fat milk and milk products. In addition, many baked goods and fried foods contain high levels of saturated fat. Even though most vegetable oils contain more unsaturated fat, there are a few that contain more saturated fat. Foods that contain coconut or coconut oil, or palm and palm kernel oils are high in saturated fats, but they do not contain cholesterol.

You can reduce your intake of saturated fats by using unsaturated fat sources (such as olive oil instead of butter or hydrogenated margarines), limiting or avoiding high-fat sauces, choosing leaner cuts of meat, avoiding processed meats, and consuming fat-free or low-fat dairy products. You should also check ingredient lists on food labels for both the amount of saturated fat in the product and for ingredients to avoid such as hydrogenated vegetable oil, shortening, coconut oil, palm kernel oil, or cocoa butter.

TO YOUR HEALTH

Just a small reduction in saturated fat can go a long way. A report by the National Cholesterol Education Program recognized that a 1 percent decrease in dietary saturated fat led to a 2 percent decrease in LDL (bad) cholesterol, which led to a 2 percent decrease in heart disease risk.

Trans Fats

The worst fat you could add to your diet would be trans fat. These types of fats are created when a liquid vegetable oil is made more solid by the addition of hydrogen through a process called *hydrogenation*. These more solid fats gained popularity with manufacturers because they increase the shelf life and flavor of many baked and processed foods.

Trans fats have received more attention lately because researchers are finding out just how dangerous they can be to health. Trans fats raise LDL (bad) cholesterol and lower your HDL (good) cholesterol. In fact, some experts believe they can raise LDL cholesterol even more than saturated fats can. Consuming these fats will increase your risk for heart disease and stroke and is also associated with a higher risk for developing type 2 diabetes.

HEALTHY MORSELS

In January 2006, the FDA required that all manufacturers begin adding trans fat to their Nutrition Facts Panel on food labels to make it easier for consumers to know just how much trans fat they are eating. With this change, many manufacturers began taking trans fats out of their products. However, if the trans fat has been removed, it has most likely been replaced with another type of unhealthy fat, such as saturated fat.

Though a small amount of trans fats are found naturally in animal foods and dairy products, most are added to foods through hydrogenation. Trans fats are found in a large variety of foods including fried foods, commercial baked goods, stick margarines, shortening, fast food, snack foods, and any food that contains hydrogenated vegetable oils.

Most experts agree: the less trans fat you eat, the better. The American Heart Association recommends limiting the amount of trans fat you consume to less than 1 percent of your total daily calories. If you need 2,000 calories per day, that means getting no more than 20 of those calories from trans fats—which is 2 grams or fewer a day. You can decrease the amount of trans fats you eat by including more fruits, vegetables, whole grains, and fat-free or low-fat dairy products. Also include leaner cuts of meat, poultry without the skin, fish, seafood, legumes, nuts, and seeds. Limit your intake of commercial baked goods, crackers, cookies, and snack foods. Use olive oil over butter or margarine. Check labels for the amount of trans fat and look on ingredient lists for hydrogenated vegetable oils. Most importantly, follow the Mediterranean diet and trans fat will be a distant thought.

GOOD TO KNOW

Even products that claim to be "trans fat free" can have up to 0.5 grams of trans fat per serving by labeling law definitions. This can add up quickly, especially if you are eating more than one serving. Even if the label states "trans fat free," take a look at the ingredient list to look for *partially hydrogenated oil* to see if the product really contains any trans fats.

Dietary Cholesterol

Cholesterol in foods is not really a fat, but a fatlike substance found only in animal foods such as meat, eggs, cheese, milk, and poultry. While we do get cholesterol from the foods we eat, our liver produces all we need—so no dietary cholesterol needed. Cholesterol does play an important role in the body, but it is when we have excess that problems occur. Our body needs cholesterol for some very important functions, including making hormones, bile acids, and vitamin D. In addition, cholesterol is part of every body cell. Any unused excess cholesterol, whether from food or produced by our body, gets stored as plaque in the arteries, increasing the risk for heart disease and stroke. Therefore limiting dietary cholesterol and the fats that raise blood cholesterol—saturated fats and trans fats—is part of the heart-healthy equation.

For people who already have high cholesterol, therapeutic diet guidelines can include as much as 10 percent of total calories from polyunsaturated fats and up to 20 percent from monounsaturated fats, since these fats can actually help to lower blood cholesterol levels and the risk for heart disease. This explains a lot when it comes to the Mediterranean diet—it's high in both of these unsaturated fats and therefore is a heart-healthy diet.

Replacing Unhealthy Fats with Healthy Ones

Although most of us realize that too much of the wrong types of fat can be dangerous to our health, we live in an overweight society that continues to get bigger and more unhealthy. We may know what we should and shouldn't eat, but making it part of our everyday lifestyle is a struggle. The most crucial strategy to remember is that you should not only add healthy fats to your diet but also replace the unhealthy fats with the healthy fats. Replacing unhealthy fats with healthier fats doesn't need to be a huge change; from a health standpoint, it is worth the modification. Even small changes can add up to big benefits. There are many ways to reduce the bad fat and increase the good fat. Following the Mediterranean diet will ensure you are on the right track. Here are a few strategies to help you get started:

- Create your own salad dressings instead of using commercial dressings that can often be overly processed and full of saturated fats. Mix olive oil with your favorite herbs and spices for a quick and healthy dressing.

- Throw out the butter and margarine and substitute olive oil or canola oil to use on bread, vegetables, and pasta or in recipes.

- Replace some of the fat in baked goods with applesauce or other puréed fruit. Use canola oil or light or extra-light olive oil for baking cakes or muffins.

- Choose fat-free (skim) milk over whole milk or low-fat milk. Fat-free milk has all of the same nutrients as whole milk minus the saturated fat.

- Choose leaner cuts of meat and eat moderate portions. Choose fish and vegetarian dishes more often.

- Read food labels and toss, or do not purchase, foods with partially hydrogenated oils or ones that contain trans fats on the Nutrition Facts Panel.

- When eating out, don't be afraid to ask the server what type of oil they use in their cooking. If you are not sure, do not order anything cooked in fat.

- Try using low-fat yogurt to replace sour cream in recipes or baking.

- Replace one egg with two egg whites in recipes to cut back on fat and cholesterol.

The Least You Need to Know

- Fats are necessary for our health and have important functions in the body.
- The Mediterranean diet is high in healthy monounsaturated fats found in olive oil, nuts, and seeds.
- The Mediterranean diet is also high in omega-3 fatty acids, a healthy polyunsaturated fat found in fish, seafood, nuts, and seeds.
- Most diets are too high in omega-6 fatty acids and too low in omega-3 fatty acids. The Mediterranean diet boasts a healthy balance.
- Saturated fats and trans fats are unhealthy fats and should be limited as much as possible. The Mediterranean diet contains very little of these unhealthy fats.
- The key to a healthy diet is not only adding healthy fats to your diet but also replacing the unhealthy ones already there.

Fill Up on Fiber

In This Chapter

- Explaining fiber
- Soluble or insoluble, all fiber is healthy
- Fiber and its benefits
- The Mediterranean diet delivers
- How much is enough?
- Increasing fiber the Mediterranean way

Do you need to lower your cholesterol, need relief from persistent constipation, want to lower your risk for certain cancers, or need to get blood sugars in check? If you answered yes to any of these questions, then your solution just might be a high-fiber diet like the Mediterranean diet. The cuisine of the Mediterranean is known for its fiber-rich content, and fiber is known to help in all of those situations. Following the diet patterns of the Mediterranean will all but guarantee you get the fiber that your body needs for optimal health in a tasty and nutritious way.

What Is Fiber?

You have heard that the Mediterranean diet is chock-full of fiber, but now you need to find out exactly what it is. Fiber is the substance found in plant cell walls that gives plants their shape and structure. You may also have heard of fiber being referred to as *roughage* or *bulk*. Our bodies cannot digest or absorb fiber, so it basically comes in and goes out while performing some amazing feats on its travels.

Dietary fiber, or the fiber found in foods, is referred to as a complex carbohydrate, but because it doesn't provide nutritional value it's not considered a nutrient. However, you can still find it listed on food nutrient labels to help you identify foods rich in fiber.

HEALTHY MORSELS

Although fiber falls under the carbohydrate category, don't let this confuse you. It does not provide the same number of calories as other carbohydrates nor is it processed in the body the same way other sources of carbohydrates are.

Breaking Down Fiber

Not all fiber is created equal. Fiber is broken down into two categories: *soluble* and *insoluble*. They differ in their abilities to dissolve in water as well as their health effects on the body. However, one is not better than the other. In fact, they are both important to our health; the key is to eat a variety of fiber-rich foods each day in order to get enough of both types of fiber. Many foods contain both types of fiber, although some may predominantly contain one type of fiber over the other.

Soluble Fiber

Soluble fiber dissolves in water. These fibers include pectins, gums, and mucilages to name a few. Soluble fibers help lower bad blood cholesterol levels, which in turn can help reduce your risk for heart disease. The people of the Mediterranean regions have a very low incidence of and risk for heart disease. In addition, this amazing fiber can help to slow down the rate at which glucose (blood sugar) is absorbed by the body. This may help control blood sugar levels in people with diabetes and other blood sugar problems.

The following foods contain generous quantities of soluble fiber:

- Legumes such as pinto beans, lima beans, navy beans, and soybeans
- Barley
- Fruits such as apricots, apples, pears, red currants, and grapes
- Vegetables such as artichokes, beets, carrots, cauliflower, and broccoli
- Seeds such as flaxseed, sesame seeds, and sunflower seeds

Insoluble Fiber

Insoluble fibers do not dissolve in water. These fibers are the ones better known as roughage and include cellulose, hemicellulose, and lignan. Insoluble fibers help move things down the intestinal tract and soften stools, helping you to avoid constipation. In addition to promoting regularity, these mighty fibers may help to decrease your risk for colon cancer, hemorrhoids, and a condition known as *diverticulosis*.

DEFINITION

Diverticulosis is a condition of the colon in which tiny pouches, or diverticula, form on the colon walls. Many times no symptoms are present until these pouches become infected or inflamed. When this takes place the condition is known as diverticulitis.

The following foods contain generous quantities of insoluble fiber:

- Whole-grain breads and cereals
- Wheat bran
- Brown rice
- Nuts such as almonds, hazelnuts, and walnuts
- Seeds such as flaxseed and sesame seeds
- Legumes such as lentils, soybeans, white beans, kidney beans, and peanuts
- Fruits such as avocados, dates, grapes, cherries, and berries
- Vegetables such as dark green leafy vegetables, eggplant, onions, and broccoli

Fiber's Healthy Benefits

Unlike some nutrients out there, your life doesn't rely on fiber for survival. However, your overall health just might. Not only do fiber's special benefits promote good health but they may also help reduce the risk for some chronic health conditions. Fiber hardly works alone, though. Most foods that include a significant amount of fiber also supply essential nutrients such as complex carbohydrates, vitamins, minerals, antioxidants, and phytonutrients—so it seems to be a package deal!

Increase Your Heart Health

Ever since Dr. Ancel Keys published his ever-popular Seven Countries Study in the 1950s, much attention was given to the fact that people from the Mediterranean regions experienced the lowest percentages of mortality from cardiovascular diseases. Something obviously needed to be said about the way these folks ate. A Mediterranean diet pattern consists of a wide variety of foods high in fiber and low in saturated fat, both of which are important for managing risk factors associated with heart disease.

There are many components that lead to heart health, so why is fiber so special? A fiber-rich diet, especially rich in soluble fiber, has the ability to help lower total blood cholesterol levels—more specifically, LDL (bad) cholesterol. Soluble fiber binds with cholesterol, which keeps it from becoming reabsorbed and instead pulls it out of the body as waste. Lowering your total cholesterol can mean lowering your risk for heart and artery disease. Recent data also suggests that adequate fiber intake can lower blood pressure as well. Want yet another heart-healthy benefit? Higher-fiber foods will, with any luck, displace your high-fat foods in meals and snacks, lowering your overall fat intake—a double bonus!

The Mediterranean diet differs from many others in that meals revolve around plant foods that are naturally high in fiber as opposed to animal foods, which can contribute loads of saturated fat and cholesterol—both of which can lead to heart disease. That's not to say that animal foods are not part of this eating style, but they play a much smaller role than plant-based foods. In addition, the animal foods that are included are much lower in saturated fat and cholesterol. Popular Mediterranean foods and dishes such as lentil soup, hummus, bulgur, and tabbouleh are high in fiber and low in saturated fat and cholesterol, a winning combination for good heart health.

Manage Your Waistline

We have long known that there is a strong correlation between a healthy body weight and the Mediterranean diet. Many factors may be at work here, but—believe it or not—fiber is truly one of the main explanations.

Fiber-rich foods such as fruits, vegetables, legumes, and whole grains can help make you feel fuller sooner, helping you to eat less. In addition, they can help keep you satisfied longer, keeping you from nibbling when you shouldn't. Fewer calories mean less fat on the hips! That might explain why many people use the Mediterranean diet not only for better health but also to drop a few extra pounds.

Keep in mind that fiber alone isn't the magic cure for weight loss. Those healthy, high-fiber foods need to replace foods high in calories, fat, and sugar. As with most of the health benefits associated with fiber, you will get the most bang for your buck if you incorporate your higher-fiber diet with a healthy, well-balanced diet and an active lifestyle.

Control Your Blood Sugar

With its fiber-rich components, the Mediterranean diet has been shown to protect against type 2 diabetes. Obese or overweight folks are prone to developing type 2 diabetes, so it makes sense that if the Mediterranean diet can help to manage waistlines, then it can protect against type 2 diabetes in that way. But even more importantly, for people with type 2 diabetes or other blood sugar ailments, a diet high in fiber (especially soluble fiber) can be a major advantage. Fiber seems to help slow the absorption of sugar into the bloodstream, which in turn slows down the rise of glucose or blood sugar. For some people this can help reduce the need for medications. However, if you have diabetes or other blood sugar problems, be sure to speak with your doctor or a dietitian before using a fiber-rich diet to control your blood sugar levels.

HEALTHY MORSELS

A 2007 study published in the *Journal of Nutritional Biochemistry* states that there are several mechanistic links that may offer a possible explanation of the Mediterranean diet's protective effect against obesity and type 2 diabetes. One such link is the high consumption of fruits, vegetables, legumes, nuts, and cereals that lead to a high consumption of dietary fiber.

Reduce Your Risk for Colon Cancer

Research shows strong evidence that a diet rich in fiber can help to lower your chance of developing colon and rectal cancers. How, you ask? By speeding up the time it takes for waste to move through your digestive tract, it leaves less time for cancer-causing agents to hang around and come in contact with the intestinal walls. In addition, fiber helps to form a bulkier, heavier stool and controls the pH balance or the level of acidity and alkalinity within the intestines.

Because most high-fiber diets are lower in saturated fats, this also may provide protection. Saturated fats have a strong correlation with the risk for colon cancer.

So again, your diet needs not only to be higher in fiber, but it needs to be the whole package (like the Mediterranean diet) to reap all of the benefits.

Support Your Digestive Health

Because the Mediterranean diet is rich in fiber, it can help you to dodge some uncomfortable and sometimes painful flare-ups from digestive disorders such as diverticulosis. A higher-fiber diet is used as standard therapy for folks who are diagnosed with diverticular disease of the colon, which can lead to symptoms such as abdominal pain, fever, and diarrhea. Softer and more regular bowel movements can also prevent constipation and the discomfort that comes with it. In addition, softer and bulkier stools can help to decrease your chance of developing hemorrhoids. All these benefits come from following a diet high in fiber!

How Much Fiber Do You Need?

The daily needs of fiber differ for men and women, and they change as we age. At this time there is no RDA (Recommended Daily Allowance) for fiber; however, there is what is termed an AI or Adequate Intake. The American Dietetic Association has found that the average American consumes only about 15 grams of fiber daily, which is well below the recommended levels and well below the intake of people in the Mediterranean regions.

According to the National Academy of Sciences Institute of Medicine, daily AI for women 50 years and younger is 25 grams; for women 51 and older, 21 grams. For men 50 years and younger, the daily AI is 38 grams; for men 51 years and older, 30 grams. Children's needs are estimated differently. A simple way to determine recommended grams of fiber for a child older than 2 years is to add 5 to the child's age in years. For example, a 5-year-old should get about 10 grams of fiber daily. After the age of 15, daily needs should be as recommended above.

Tips to Increase Your Fiber Intake

It really isn't as hard as you may think to increase your daily fiber intake. Following some easy tips that coincide with the Mediterranean diet can sneak plenty of fiber into your daily plan. It is all about healthy habits and making permanent lifestyle changes.

GOOD TO KNOW

Be careful to ease your body into a higher-fiber diet. You should increase fiber gradually over several weeks to help your body adjust to the change. Too much fiber too quickly could result in some uncomfortable symptoms such as bloating, gas, and cramping.

Increase your fluid intake with a higher-fiber diet. Fiber acts as a bulking agent, soaking up some of the fluids in your body. Therefore it is important to drink extra fluid to keep from becoming dehydrated. More importantly, additional fluids will help to keep that fiber traveling to where it needs to go!

Follow these simple tips to help you increase your daily fiber intake:

- Try dried fruits which are usually higher in fiber than fresh fruit.

- Switch your white bread to breads that are made with 100 percent whole grain. Be sure to check the label to ensure you have a whole-grain product.

- Experiment with popular fiber-rich grains of the Mediterranean such as bulgur. Bulgur is very versatile and can be used as a meat extender or as a meat substitute in meatless meals. It can also be used in place of rice or couscous in your favorite dishes.

- Try adding legumes such as fava beans, lentils, or white beans to your meals a few times a week. They offer loads of fiber and protein. Give them a try in soups, stews, casseroles, or salads.

- Stock your pantry with brown rice and whole-wheat pasta or couscous instead of their white counterparts.

- Leave the skin or peel on fruits and vegetables when possible and wash them well before eating. Most of the fiber found in fruits and vegetables is found in the skin and pulp.

- When you feel the urge to snack, grab a piece of fresh or dried fruit, a handful of nuts, or a few tablespoons of seeds.

- Eat whole fruits and vegetables more often than juices. Most of the fiber found in fruits and veggies is removed when the juice is produced.

Label Fiber Lingo

Now you know that fresh produce, dried fruits, nuts, and beans are naturally good sources of fiber. But what about breads, cereals, pastas, crackers, and other grains? Finding those may take a little more knowledge and practice. To take the mystery out of finding high-fiber foods, you need to learn how to decipher the food label:

- **Good Source of Fiber:** contains 2.5 to 4.9 grams per serving, or 10 to 19 Percent Daily Value

- **High in Fiber, Rich in Fiber, or Excellent Source of Fiber:** contains 5 grams or more per serving, or 20 Percent Daily Value

- **More or Added Fiber:** contains at least 2.5 grams more per serving than the reference food

Don't Overdo It!

You *can* get too much of a good thing by overdoing your fiber intake. Although enough fiber is vital to good health, too much fiber can cause some uncomfortable side effects such as diarrhea, gas, bloating, and cramping. Excessive amounts of fiber, in the range of 50 grams or more each day, can also reduce the absorption of some very important nutrients such as zinc, calcium, magnesium, and iron. The key is to stay in the recommended range of fiber intake for your age and gender. Gradually increase your fiber daily over a period of several weeks to get your body adjusted to it, and drink plenty of fluids as well. This will ensure you get the fiber you need and that your body can handle it without any adverse effects.

GOOD TO KNOW

The market is stocked with fiber supplements. To get all of the benefits that fiber provides, don't take the easy way out. Whole foods provide more fiber as well as added essential nutrients such as vitamins, minerals, antioxidants, and phytonutrients that are necessary for optimal health. Never replace whole foods or any food group with a simple supplement.

How the Mediterranean Diet Delivers High Fiber

People of the Mediterranean lean toward including fiber-rich foods at every meal and snack. Meals revolve around vegetables, nuts, and beans instead of meat, and desserts chiefly consist of fruits or nuts. Whole grains are used instead of refined grains, and processed foods are used very minimally. All of these points equal one fiber-rich diet. The foods highest in fiber are listed in the following table as a handy reference.

Fiber-Rich Foods

Vegetables	Grams of Fiber
Artichoke hearts, cooked ($\frac{1}{2}$ cup)	7.2
Peas, green, cooked ($\frac{1}{2}$ cup)	4.4
Tomato, sun-dried ($\frac{1}{2}$ cup)	3.3
Red potato, baked, with skin (1 medium)	2.5
Spinach, cooked ($\frac{1}{2}$ cup)	2.2
Broccoli, cooked ($\frac{1}{2}$ cup)	2.6
Cabbage, cooked ($\frac{1}{2}$ cup)	1.9
Carrots, raw, chopped ($\frac{1}{2}$ cup)	1.8
Mushrooms, cooked ($\frac{1}{2}$ cup)	1.7
Turnips, cooked ($\frac{1}{2}$ cup)	1.6
Tomato, raw, 1 medium	1.5
Onions, raw, chopped ($\frac{1}{2}$ cup)	1.4
Cauliflower, cooked ($\frac{1}{2}$ cup)	1.4
Eggplant, cooked ($\frac{1}{2}$ cup)	1.25

Fruits	Grams of Fiber
Avocados, (1 fruit)	9.2
Raspberries, raw (1 cup)	8.0
Prunes (1 cup)	7.7
Blueberries, raw (1 cup)	7.6
Dates, chopped ($\frac{1}{2}$ cup)	5.9
Figs, dried ($\frac{1}{2}$ cup)	5.5

continues

Fiber-Rich Foods   (continued)

Fruits	Grams of Fiber
Raisins, seedless (1 cup)	5.4
Pear, raw, with skin (1 medium)	5.1
Apple, raw, with skin (1 medium)	3.3
Strawberries, raw (1 cup)	3.3
Apricots, raw, sliced (1 cup)	3.3

Grains, Cereal, Pasta	Grams of Fiber
Whole-wheat pasta, cooked (1 cup)	6.3
Barley, pearled, cooked (1 cup)	6.0
Bulgur, cooked ($\frac{1}{2}$ cup)	4.1
Brown rice, long-grain, cooked (1 cup)	3.5
Quinoa, cooked ($\frac{1}{2}$ cup)	2.6
Couscous, cooked ($\frac{1}{2}$ cup)	1.1
Whole-wheat bread (1 slice)	1.9
Wheat germ (1 TB.)	1.1

Legumes, Nuts, Seeds	Grams of Fiber
Split peas, cooked ($\frac{1}{2}$ cup)	8.2
Lentils, cooked ($\frac{1}{2}$ cup)	7.8
Black beans, cooked ($\frac{1}{2}$ cup)	7.5
Lima beans, cooked ($\frac{1}{2}$ cup)	6.6
Kidney beans, cooked ($\frac{1}{2}$ cup)	6.5
Chickpeas, cooked ($\frac{1}{2}$ cup)	6.25
White beans, cooked ($\frac{1}{2}$ cup)	5.6
Fava beans (or broad beans), cooked ($\frac{1}{2}$ cup)	4.6
Almonds (1 oz.)	3.5
Peanuts (1 oz.)	2.4
Walnuts (1 oz.)	1.9

Source: USDA National Nutrient Database for Standard Reference, Release 22, 2009;
www.ars.usda.gov

Fiber Intake the Mediterranean Way

To prove how simple a day in the life on the Mediterranean diet might be, here is a sample (see Chapter 23 for more seasonal menu plans that help increase your fiber):

- Breakfast might include sliced tomato or cucumber with a soft cheese such as feta, goat cheese, or mozzarella; fresh fruit; whole-wheat toast, pita bread, or flatbread dipped in olive oil; or low-fat or fat-free plain or Greek yogurt.

- Snacks might include fresh fruit; a handful of nuts or seeds; a piece of soft cheese; whole-grain crackers; or low-fat or fat-free plain or Greek yogurt flavored with honey.

- Lunch might include a bean or lentil soup; a salad made with plenty of greens, fresh vegetables, and olives; and fresh fruit.

- Dinner might include a stew made with poultry, fish, or shellfish; a whole grain such as brown rice or couscous; steamed fresh vegetables drizzled with olive oil; fresh fruit; and a small glass of red wine.

TO YOUR HEALTH

Cooking your vegetables too much can reduce their fiber content. When cooking veggies, try steaming them or cooking them quickly in the microwave.

Fiber Up Your Favorite Foods the Mediterranean Way

Fiber up your cooking methods by substituting whole-wheat flour in baked goods or adding wheat bran or oat bran to stews, casseroles, muffins, or yogurt. Try using brown rice or whole-grain couscous instead of white rice or substituting whole-wheat pasta for regular pasta in your favorite recipes.

Take zucchini, for example. It can be as easy as to prepare zucchini and add mushrooms, pine nuts, onions, a pinch of mint, and a splash of olive oil. You have just turned plain zucchini into a wonderfully tasty Mediterranean dish, full of extra fiber, healthy fats, and loads of other essential nutrients. The possibilities are endless.

The Least You Need to Know

- Fiber is a type of carbohydrate that is an indigestible part of plants.
- Fiber-rich foods include fruits, vegetables, whole grains, nuts, seeds, and beans.
- Evidence suggests that soluble and insoluble fiber help to lower the risk for heart disease and cancer, control blood sugar, and promote regularity.
- The Mediterranean diet delivers loads of fiber-rich foods that contribute to its many health benefits.

Nutrients in the Mediterranean Diet

In This Chapter

- Mediterranean foods pack in the nutrients
- The small but mighty nutrients
- Never underestimate an antioxidant
- The more color, the better
- More macronutrients

With all of the healthy foods included on the Mediterranean diet, it's not surprising to discover just how jam-packed it is with a vast array of nutrients. The Mediterranean diet has been cited in many clinical papers as being heart healthy and an all-around healthy diet. What is it about nutrients such as vitamins, minerals, antioxidants, and phytonutrients that make this style of eating so much healthier? You need to become familiar with these nutrients to get a better understanding of the complete nutritional package of the Mediterranean diet.

Nutrients of Mediterranean Foods

There are 13 main food groups that are included in the Mediterranean diet: whole grains, fruits, vegetables, low-fat and fat-free dairy foods, seafood, poultry, olives, legumes, nuts and seeds, potatoes, eggs, some lean red meats, and olive oil, as well as red wine. All of these foods contribute an abundance of essential nutrients, and study after study proves that the nutrients that make up the Mediterranean diet boost health and longevity. (See Part 2 to review some of the more common foods on the Mediterranean diet and find information on their micronutrient and phytonutrient contents.)

TO YOUR HEALTH

Curious about the nutritional content of some other favorite Mediterranean foods? Check out the USDA's Food Database at www.nal.usda.gov/fnic/foodcomp/search.

The Almighty Vitamins

Vitamins are organic compounds and a group of nutrients that are required in small, even tiny, amounts for optimal health. This earned them the name *micronutrients*. But don't let the *micro* part fool you. They have big jobs and are involved in just about every function your body performs, from helping fat, protein, and carbohydrates to supply energy to regulating body processes. Some of these vitamins can be obtained from synthesis in the body; however, most are essential, and we need to get them from the foods we eat. A balanced diet can provide just about all of the vitamins our body needs. Now you can start to appreciate just why our diet and the food we put into our bodies is so incredibly important!

It's easy to get confused about all the vitamins out there, so let's try to simplify it. There are 13 essential vitamins that are needed for our body to function properly, and these are subdivided into two groups: fat-soluble and water-soluble vitamins. Their categories explain how they are both carried in food and transported in the body.

HEALTHY MORSELS

Contrary to what you may have heard, vitamins do not supply energy directly, but they do regulate and are needed for the breakdown or metabolism of carbs, proteins, and fats that directly supply energy to our body.

Fat-Soluble Vitamins

Fat-soluble vitamins dissolve in fat, and that's how they are carried through the bloodstream and the body. It's one reason we do need moderate amounts of fat in our diet. Fat-soluble vitamins can be stored in fat tissue and the liver, and concentrations can build up over time. Therefore, you don't want to consume excessive amounts of fat-soluble vitamins for long periods, as that can be harmful. The fat-soluble vitamins are:

- **Vitamin A:** Promotes normal vision and the growth and health of body cells and tissue, regulates our immune system, and works as an antioxidant in the form of carotenoids. Too much vitamin A in the form of supplements can be toxic to your body, because it can be stored. However, eating lots of foods rich in beta-carotene, even though it turns into vitamin A, is not toxic because the body converts beta-carotene into vitamin A only when we need it. Vitamin A is found in liver, milk, fortified breakfast cereals, and eggs. Beta-carotene is found in orange, red, yellow, and dark green veggies and fruits (such as carrots and cantaloupe); sweet potatoes; and spinach.

- **Vitamin D:** Essential for the absorption of calcium and phosphorus and for depositing them in the bones and teeth to help make them strong. Vitamin D is also responsible for the regulation of cell growth and for protecting the immune system. The body can make its own vitamin D when the skin is exposed to moderate amounts of sunlight for short periods of time. New research is uncovering even more benefits of vitamin D, which include heart health, lowering blood pressure, and longevity. Vitamin D is found in fortified milk, cereals, and juices; eggs; and fish oils (salmon, shrimp, canned sardines, and cod).

- **Vitamin E:** Aids in the formation and functioning of red blood cells and other tissues, acts as a powerful antioxidant to protect essential fatty acids, and prevents cell damage from free radicals—all of which may help to lower the risk for heart disease, stroke, cancer, and other health conditions of aging. Vitamin E is found in vegetable oils; olives; almonds and hazelnuts; sunflower seeds; peanuts; whole grains, fortified cereals; green leafy vegetables (spinach, mustard greens, turnip greens, kale, chard); and fruits and vegetables such as bell peppers, kiwis, tomatoes, blueberries, and broccoli.

GOOD TO KNOW

Vegetable oils, including extra-virgin olive oil, are a good source of vitamin E, so people who cut back too much on fat may not get enough.

- **Vitamin K:** Aids in the regulation of blood clotting to help bleeding stop. The body can produce vitamin K from certain bacteria in the intestines, but we also get it from foods. Vitamin K is found in green leafy vegetables (spinach, chard, kale, mustard greens); Brussels sprouts, green beans, asparagus, cauliflower, broccoli, green peas, and carrots; soybeans and black-eyed peas; and pine nuts and pistachios.

Water-Soluble Vitamins

Water-soluble vitamins dissolve in water and are carried through the body by watery fluids. Most water-soluble vitamins are not stored in the body, at least not in significant amounts. Instead the body uses what it needs and excretes the rest through urine. Because this group of vitamins isn't stored, you need a constant supply from your diet to make sure you have optimal amounts. There is less worry of toxicity with water-soluble vitamins but more worry of deficiency. The water-soluble vitamins are:

- **Vitamin C:** Boosts the immune system, produces collagen to hold bones and muscles together, keeps blood vessels healthy, helps to absorb iron, aids in wound healing, produces healthy gums, helps to protect from infection, and acts as an antioxidant. Sources include citrus fruits, berries, peppers, potatoes, green leafy vegetables, and tomatoes.

- **Folate (Folic Acid):** Essential for cell division and red blood cell production, helps to produce DNA (our genetic makeup), may help protect against heart disease, and has the ability to reduce neural tube birth defects in newborns. Sources include dark green leafy vegetables, avocados, peanuts, most beans, lentils, oranges, fortified breakfast cereals, and wheat germ.

- **Thiamin (B_1):** Needed to convert carbohydrate-containing foods into energy and helps keep the brain, nervous system, and heart cells healthy. Sources include lean pork, whole grains, legumes, oatmeal, seeds, spinach, lamb, and lean beef.

- **Riboflavin (B_2):** Helps produce energy from protein, fat, and carbs; assists in the formation of red blood cells; maintains healthy skin, nails, hair, and normal vision. Sources include yogurt and milk, eggs, whole-grain breads and cereals, cheese, green leafy vegetables, oysters, and clams.

- **Niacin (B_3):** Helps the body utilize sugars and fatty acids for energy; produces energy in all body cells; maintains normal enzyme function; maintains healthy skin, nerves, and digestion. Sources include lean meats and poultry, seafood, nuts, brown rice, milk, eggs, enriched breads and cereals, whole grains, legumes, and green vegetables.

- **Pyridoxine (B_6):** Helps make nonessential amino acids (building blocks of protein) which are then used to make body cells; maintains normal brain function; and aids in formation of insulin, red blood cells, and antibodies. Sources include lean meats and poultry, legumes, whole grains, seafood, lentils, green leafy vegetables, carrots, peas, corn, bananas, mangos, potatoes, milk, cheese, and eggs.

- **Cobalamin (B$_{12}$):** Helps in the formation of red blood cells, helps the body to utilize fatty acids and some amino acids, maintains healthy nerve cells, and is needed to make DNA genetic material. Sources include lean meats and poultry, seafood, eggs, and milk products.

- **Pantothenic Acid and Biotin:** Involved in the metabolism and production of energy from proteins, fats, and carbohydrates and is essential for growth. Sources include eggs, seafood, milk products, whole grains, legumes, potatoes, lean beef, and vegetables in the cabbage family (such as broccoli).

GOOD TO KNOW

Do not rely solely on dietary supplements to provide your daily allotment of vitamins and minerals. Dietary supplements provide only what is listed on the bottle and omit phytonutrients, fiber, and other natural substances that have been proven to be health-promoting. As a rule of thumb: food before pills. Supplements should *supplement* your diet, not be used as replacements for foods or food groups. They will not make up for a poor diet.

The Mighty Minerals

Minerals are one mighty bunch of essential nutrients needed to regulate a host of body processes that are continually taking place—basically, they make things happen. Minerals have myriad jobs including giving structure to your body by building strong bones, regulating fluid balance, aiding in muscle contractions, and transmitting nerve impulses. In addition, some minerals are used to make hormones and maintain a normal heartbeat. Unlike vitamins, minerals are inorganic and much tougher. They cannot be destroyed by heat or food-handling methods like vitamins can. Minerals are first absorbed into the intestines. Some pass directly into the bloodstream and then onto cells, with excess being excreted in the urine. Others are carried by attaching to proteins and become a part of the body's structure. Because these types are stored, excess amounts over long periods of time can be harmful.

Not all minerals have a Recommended Dietary Allowance (RDA) that has been set. Minerals that do have an RDA include copper, iodine, iron, molybdenum, selenium, and zinc. The others have Adequate Intake (AI) levels instead.

Minerals come in two categories: major and trace, as detailed in the following table. Major minerals are needed by the body in greater amounts than trace minerals. It doesn't mean one is any more important than the other, just that the body needs varying amounts to do its job.

Major Minerals	Trace Minerals
Calcium	Chromium
Chloride	Cobalt
Magnesium	Copper
Phosphorus	Fluoride
Potassium	Iodine
Sodium	Iron
Sulfur	Manganese
	Molybdenum
	Selenium
	Zinc

A few other minerals, including boron, nickel, arsenic, silicon, and vanadium, have not yet been deemed necessary for health by nutrition experts.

Both major and trace minerals are essential for many vital bodily functions and processes. Minerals are abundant and can be found in a wide variety of foods that are common to the Mediterranean diet. However, we will focus on just a few of the powerhouse players:

- **Calcium:** Calcium is the most abundant mineral in our body with almost 99 percent of it being stored in the tissues of the bones. In addition to giving bones strength, this major mineral helps to slow the rate of bone loss as you age, helps muscles to contract and the heart to beat, regulates blood pressure, regulates normal nerve function, helps blood to clot if you are bleeding, and helps keep teeth strong and healthy. If you don't get enough calcium in your diet, your bones will release stored calcium into your blood and weakened bones will result. Sources include milk and most dairy products, canned sardines and salmon with edible bones, broccoli, legumes, almonds, dried figs, dark green leafy vegetables such as spinach and kale, calcium-fortified tofu, and other fortified foods such as orange juice.

- **Iron:** A good part of this mineral can be found in your red blood cells, also known as *hemoglobin*. It serves as a delivery service, transporting oxygen from your lungs throughout the body to where it is needed. Iron is also necessary for brain development and for a healthy immune system. If you don't get enough iron, you don't get enough oxygen to the rest of your body. That can result in anemia, which can show up as fatigue, weakness, headaches, irritability, and the feeling of being cold. Iron is found in a variety of food sources, including lean red meats, poultry, pork, lamb, veal, fish, oysters, clams, egg yolks, legumes, lentils, whole grains, dark green leafy vegetables, dried fruits, nuts and seeds, fortified cereals, and wheat germ.

- **Selenium:** Working with vitamin E, selenium acts as a powerful antioxidant to protect cells from damage that may lead to heart disease, cancer, and other chronic health conditions. It aids in cell growth and boosts immune function. Sources of selenium include lean meats, eggs, wheat germ, garlic, whole grains, Brazil nuts, walnuts, peanuts, sunflower seeds, raisins, shellfish (lobster, oysters, shrimp, scallops), and fish (salmon, tuna, mackerel, halibut, flounder, and herring). It can also be found in alfalfa, fennel seed, radish, horseradish, onion, chives, and some mushrooms.

TO YOUR HEALTH

How much you need of both vitamins and minerals depends on your age, gender, and current health status. Check out the whole list of DRIs (Dietary Reference Intakes) for all vitamins and minerals at fnic.nal.usda.gov.

The Role of Antioxidants

You've heard the word *antioxidants* pop up a lot in this book. Antioxidants are a group of nutrients that counteract effects of harmful free radicals. Free radicals can come from the environment and include things like cigarette smoke, pollution, and ultraviolet light. But these free radicals are also produced as a by-product of the oxygen that our very own body cells burn (oxidation). These free radicals created by oxidation of cells are unstable and can damage body cells, tissues, and DNA, causing all sorts of health issues including heart and artery disease, cancer, cataracts, age-related disorders such as diabetes and Alzheimer's disease, and general age-related deterioration. The cells in our body have their own natural defenses against free radicals, but research has discovered that certain vitamins, minerals, and phytonutrients can also help ward off the effect of and damage from these free radicals—and they are fittingly called antioxidants.

Some of the more common antioxidants include:

- Beta-carotene (which forms vitamin A in the body)
- Vitamin C
- Vitamin E
- Selenium

Phytonutrients of the Rainbow

Foods of the Mediterranean diet are chock-full of phytonutrients. So why is that such a big deal? Unlike some of the other nutrients we have discussed (vitamins, minerals, proteins, carbohydrates, and fats) phytonutrients are not essential for human life; however, they have been found to promote good health in a very big way. There are many classes of phytonutrients and they can be grouped by color. Many of the foods high in phytonutrients are brightly colored (like fruits and vegetables), and all of the color groups boast a wide array of phytonutrients. This is exactly why we have repeated so many times that it is important to eat a variety of colorful fruits and vegetables. The more colors, the more phytonutrients!

What's All the Hype?

There is definite reason to give these relatively recent discoveries all the hype they are receiving. Phytonutrients are thought to provide health benefits that go beyond that of vitamins and minerals. For a long time, it has been evident that people, like people of the Mediterranean, who eat a lot of plant foods, including fruits and vegetables, seem to be healthier, display lower incidences of chronic diseases such as cancer and heart disease, and live longer lives. It has always been assumed that these results were the workings of essential vitamins and minerals. But it turns out that was only part of the story, and that there might just be thousands of other substances in these plant foods that are beneficial to human health. The belief is that these phytonutrients work synergistically with fiber, vitamins, minerals, and antioxidants to promote health and provide added protection. Many health organizations, including the American Heart Association and the National Cancer Institute, recommend whole foods over supplements to ensure consumption of these beneficial phytonutrients.

Discover Common Phytonutrients

Most phytonutrients are either flavonoids (which are a subclass of polyphenols) or carotenoids. Polyphenols are a broad class of phytonutrients that include not only flavonoids but also resveratrol and phenolic acids. Because there are literally thousands of phytonutrients, and more are continually being discovered and classified, we will talk about a few of the more common ones:

- **Beta-carotene (carotenoid):** Potent antioxidant to prevent damage from free radicals as well as a precursor for the formation of vitamin A. Found primarily in yellow and orange fruits and vegetables and green leafy vegetables.

- **Lutein (carotenoid):** May prevent and slow macular degeneration, a condition of the eye which can lead to blindness in the elderly. Acts as an antioxidant to prevent free radical damage to the macula of the eye, prevent formation of cataracts, reduce risk for heart disease, and protect against many types of cancer. Found primarily in green leafy vegetables including artichokes, broccoli, spinach, and kale.

- **Lycopene (carotenoid):** Potent antioxidant linked with reduced risk of cancer (especially prostate cancer) and may offer protection against heart attacks. Found primarily in red fruits and vegetables with tomato products being the most concentrated sources.

- **Anthocyanidins (flavonoid):** Linked to improved health of the blood vessels, acts as an antioxidant, and may maintain brain function and healthy immune function. Found primarily in blue, purple, and red fruits and vegetables.

Powerful Protein

So far we have discussed the micronutrients; now it's time to discover a few of the macronutrients, which consist of protein, carbs, and fat. (See Chapter 14 for a full discussion concerning fats.) Protein doesn't only come from the foods we eat but it's also part of many body structures such as collagen, muscles, bones, organs, tendons, ligaments, hair, nails, teeth, and skin. Protein is used in the body to build and repair tissues; to make enzymes and hormones; to transport nutrients; to help muscles contract; to regulate body processes such as fluid balance; and the list goes on. If you don't get enough in the way of carbohydrates, it can also be metabolized and used for energy.

There are 22 different amino acids, which we discussed in Chapter 12, that make up protein. Nine of these are essential, meaning we must get them from food, and the others come from the body's own amino acid collection. These amino acids are strung together in different combinations and make up all of the protein needed by the body for all its functions.

Is it a High-Protein Diet?

The nutrient profile of the Mediterranean diet is far from a high-protein diet. In fact, protein consists of about 15 percent of daily caloric intake, which is in line with what most health experts recommend for a healthy diet. On a typical 2,000-calorie diet, this would equate to 300 calories or 75 grams of protein. Too much protein can cause a host of health problems, so sticking with a more moderate protein intake is the way to go.

Mediterranean Protein Sources

The protein sources common to the Mediterranean diet may be a bit different than what you are used to. They include low to moderate amounts of animal proteins such as lean meats (only small amounts of red meat), dairy products, and eggs with a larger emphasis on plant protein sources such as nuts, seeds, whole grains, legumes, and lentils. Seafood is another major protein contributor. The following table lists common protein sources on the Mediterranean diet and just how much protein they contain per serving.

Mediterranean Protein Sources

Food	Protein Content*
Chicken breast, cooked (½ breast)	26.6 grams
Salmon, cooked (3 oz.)	21.6 grams
Fava beans, cooked (1 cup)	12.9 grams
Yogurt, plain, low-fat (1 cup)	12.9 grams
Lentils, cooked (½ cup)	8.9 grams
Fat-free milk (8 oz.)	8.4 grams
Eggs (1 large)	6.3 grams
Sardines (2)	5.9 grams
Bulgur, cooked (1 cup)	5.6 grams
Walnuts (1 oz.)	4.3 grams
Feta cheese (1 oz.)	4 grams

USDA National Nutrient Database for Standard Reference
www.nal.usda.gov/fnic/foodcomp/search/index.html

Energy-Boosting Mediterranean Carbs

The category of carbohydrates includes not only starches but also sugar and fiber as well. Starches and sugars are your body's main source of fuel. (You can find more on fiber in Chapter 15.) Carbohydrates can be a big source of calories in just about everyone's diet, but the type of carbohydrate you choose can make all the difference. Even though starches and sugars are both carbs, they can be very different. Sugars are considered simple carbs because they are made up of only one or two sugars. If foods have one unit of sugar they are called *monosaccharides*. These are the building blocks to *disaccharides*, which have two units of sugar. Simple sugars include foods and beverages such as honey, jelly, syrup, table sugar, candy, soft drinks, fruit juices, and yes, fruit (though fruit contains a naturally occurring sugar called fructose, not an added sugar). Even milk contains a simple, naturally occurring sugar called lactose. When you have a sweet tooth these are some of the types of carbohydrates you crave!

When three or more of these units or simple sugars are linked together, they become complex carbohydrates (or starches) and are called *polysaccharides*. Complex carbs can be found in grains, nuts, seeds, fruits, and vegetables. Foods higher in starchy complex carbs would include breads, cereal, rice, pasta, potatoes, legumes, peas, lentils, yams, winter squash, and corn. All grains include starchy carbohydrates, but whole grains are better for you because they contain more fiber and nutrient content. Complex carbs might not satisfy your sweet tooth like simple carbs because starch molecules are larger and therefore do not taste sweet.

Are Carbohydrates Okay to Eat?

No matter which type of carbohydrate we consume, simple or complex, they all are broken down to their most basic form, which is glucose. Glucose is the type of sugar or carbohydrate that is absorbed and used for energy in the body. Because simple carbs are already broken down and in a single form, they are absorbed much more quickly than complex carbs that are larger and need to be broken down more. Therefore, the longer time required to break down complex carbs means glucose is released into the bloodstream much slower than simple carbs, helping to regulate blood sugar levels. Even though fruit contains forms of simple sugars, it also contains complex carbs and fiber, and this helps to slow the absorption of glucose into the bloodstream. In addition, most purely simple carbs are empty calories meaning they provide calories but not much in the way of nutritional value, while complex carbs are quite the opposite, providing fiber and other essential nutrients. Of course, this doesn't apply to foods like fruit and milk, which both contain a form of simple sugar but are high on the nutrition content list.

HEALTHY MORSELS

If you are worried that the carbs on the Mediterranean diet will cause you to gain weight, don't be! Contrary to popular belief, carbohydrates do not make you fat and are not the lone culprit in causing people to be overweight. Eating too much, whether carbohydrates, proteins, or fats, provides excess calories that are stored as fat in the body. Glucose, or the sugar that complex carbs are broken down into, will not cause your body to make or store fat. Glucose is converted to body fat only if you consume more total calories than your body actually needs.

Carbohydrates are more than okay to eat—they are essential, and your body needs the energy that they produce. In fact, glucose is the only source of energy your brain can actually use! The key is choosing complex carbs over simple sugars, especially the empty-calorie versions. Eat carbohydrates in moderation and properly balance your diet with the other macronutrients: fat and protein.

Mediterranean Carbohydrate Sources

Carbohydrates are an essential part of any healthy diet, and as we have seen, complex carbs are a large part of the Mediterranean diet. The Mediterranean diet is made up of about 45 to 50 percent of total calories from carbohydrates, with the vast majority of these carbs coming from complex sources such as legumes, couscous, potatoes, brown rice, vegetables, barley, and bulgur, just to name a few. These are all complex carbohydrates with loads of fiber and other essential nutrients. When people of the Mediterranean eat carbs, they definitely make them count!

The Least You Need to Know

- Vitamins and minerals are essential for normal body function. Eating a varied and well-balanced diet can help you to get all your body needs.
- Vitamins are separated into water-soluble and fat-soluble categories. Minerals are either major or trace.
- Antioxidants protect from the damage of free radicals. They can help to prevent cancer, heart disease, cataracts, and a host of other chronic health conditions. The most common are beta-carotene, vitamins E and C, and selenium.

- Phytonutrients are not essential nutrients like vitamins and minerals; however, they are compounds found in plants that may work with essential nutrients to protect our health even more.
- Carbs, protein, and fat are macronutrients. Carbs are essential to a healthy diet and should consist mostly of the complex variety. Protein is moderate on the Mediterranean diet, coming more from plant sources than animal sources.

Savor the Flavors of the Mediterranean

There's nothing like delicious recipes and detailed menu plans to help inspire you to jump-start a new way of eating. The recipes and menu plans in this part of the book help you to implement this diet into your everyday life. Going to a party? No problem! You'll find plenty of appetizer recipes. Need a pizza for a Friday night supper with the family? Again, no problem—you'll find recipes to fit all of your needs and tastes. Looking for some dessert ideas that won't expand your waistline? Look no further than the delectable desserts we compile here. And after you've tried some of the recipes, check out our ideas for seasonal menu plans. Let these recipes and menus help you incorporate all the foods you have read about and are eager to try. Bon appétit!

Easy Appetizers and Snacks

In This Chapter

- Simple ingredients with big taste
- Entertaining made easy
- Tantalizing recipes

Appetizers of the Mediterranean focus on fresh, flavorful, plant-based ingredients. Mediterranean appetizers put vegetables and other plant-based foods on the A-list at any party and are the perfect way to sneak more of these nutritious foods into your diet. Appetizers of the Mediterranean aren't just extras or empty-calorie foods; they can actually be counted as servings of recommended food groups.

Delicious appetizers are all about the combinations of foods that accent and play upon each other. Ingredients are king when it comes to creating great flavor. By strategically selecting and combining a few key Mediterranean foods—such as feta cheese, sun-dried tomatoes, figs, dates, balsamic vinegar, and extra-virgin olive oil—even the most humble ingredients are elevated to appetizer greatness! One central ingredient is freshly ground black pepper, which will provide your dishes with a delightful peppery zing. You may want to consider purchasing a high-quality grinder and whole peppercorns to add a little spice to your foods.

The tantalizing recipes in this chapter span all of the seasons and use fresh, seasonal ingredients. Use the recipes in season or whenever you like!

Roasted Red Pepper Tapenade

Roasted red peppers lend a smoky-sweet flavor when blended with salty Kalamata olives for a delicious summer combination.

Yield:	Prep time:	Cook time:	Serving size:
1½ cups	15 minutes	None	2 tablespoons

Each serving has:			
15 calories	1.5 g total fat	0 g saturated fat	0 g protein
1 g carbohydrates	0 g fiber	0 mg cholesterol	70 mg sodium

2 jarred roasted red peppers, finely diced

20 pitted Kalamata olives, finely diced

1 Roma tomato, seeded and finely diced

2 cloves garlic, finely minced (about 1 tsp.)

¼ tsp. freshly ground black pepper

2 tsp. extra-virgin olive oil

1. In a medium bowl, combine roasted red peppers, olives, tomato, and garlic. Add pepper and extra-virgin olive oil. Mix well.

2. Let rest 30 minutes so flavors can meld.

3. Serve at room temperature with crackers or atop a slice of toasted baguette.

Variation: Roast your own red peppers for an even smokier flavor. Char red peppers over a gas flame or under a broiler until the skin is black all over. Place peppers in a paper bag for 10 minutes. When cool enough to handle, peel skin off peppers and discard. Slice and discard seeds and juices.

HEALTHY MORSELS

You can also use this as a sandwich spread, in an omelet, in a wrap, on a pizza, or to top chicken or fish. There are many possibilities for this versatile spread.

Pesto

Basil is the epitome of summer. Its fresh aroma is irresistible!

Yield:	Prep time:	Cook time:	Serving size:
1 cup	20 minutes	None	1 tablespoon
Each serving has:			
120 calories	12 g total fat	2.5 g saturated fat	2 g protein
1 g carbohydrates	0 g fiber	5 mg cholesterol	75 mg sodium

¼ cup pine nuts

3 cloves garlic

1 tsp. kosher salt

4 oz. fresh basil leaves (about
   3 cups packed)

⅔ cup extra-virgin olive oil

1 cup freshly grated Parmesan
   cheese

1. In a small skillet over medium heat, toast pine nuts for 5 to 6 minutes until lightly browned.

2. In a food processor, add garlic, toasted pine nuts, and salt. Process until finely chopped.

3. Add basil leaves to mixture. Process until basil is finely chopped.

4. With the food processor running, slowly add extra-virgin olive oil. Continue to process until smooth.

5. Add Parmesan cheese and pulse until cheese is incorporated. Pesto will be thick. If pesto is too thick, add 1 or 2 tablespoons of the pasta cooking water to the mixture.

Variation: Use walnuts instead of pine nuts, or try using arugula instead of basil.

TO YOUR HEALTH

You can use pesto in many ways. Mix ½ cup pesto with 1 pound pasta and serve with extra Parmesan cheese as a garnish.

Melon, Prosciutto, and Figs

Balsamic vinegar becomes sweet when reduced and is a nice contrast with the salty components in this summer dish.

Yield:	Prep time:	Cook time:	Serving size:
4 servings	15 minutes	9 minutes	¼ recipe

Each serving has:			
250 calories	14 g total fat	7 g saturated fat	11 g protein
22 g carbohydrates	2 g fiber	35 mg cholesterol	550 mg sodium

½ cup balsamic vinegar

½ cantaloupe, peeled and seeded

4 fresh figs

4 thin slices prosciutto

4 oz. goat cheese, crumbled

1 TB. extra-virgin olive oil

Freshly ground black pepper to taste

1. In a small saucepan, add balsamic vinegar and cook over high heat for 9 minutes or until liquid has reduced to 2 tablespoons. Liquid should be thick. Remove from heat and let cool.

2. Cut melon into about 24 thin slices. Each plate should have about 6 slices.

3. Slice each fig lengthwise into 4 pieces.

4. Place ¼ melon onto individual plates.

5. Roll up prosciutto from short end. Place one roll on each plate.

6. Divide sliced figs equally among the plates. Crumble 1 ounce goat cheese over each.

7. Drizzle each plate with cooled balsamic vinegar and olive oil. Sprinkle with black pepper.

Stuffed Dates

These stuffed dates are sweet and savory. If you think you don't like dates, try these for a perfect fall dish!

Yield:	Prep time:	Cook time:	Serving size:
12 dates	15 minutes	15 minutes	1 date

Each serving has:			
170 calories	5 g total fat	2 g saturated fat	4 g protein
31 g carbohydrates	3 g fiber	10 mg cholesterol	150 mg sodium

1 Italian sausage link

12 Medjool dates

3 TB. roasted almonds, finely chopped

½ cup goat cheese

2 TB. finely chopped fresh parsley

1. In a small skillet over medium heat, cook Italian sausage link for 12 to 15 minutes or until done. Remove from heat and let cool. Slice link in half lengthwise. Cut one half link crosswise into 12 half-rounds. (The other half link can be saved for another use.)

2. Slit each date down the center and remove pit. Be careful not to slice all the way through date or through the ends.

3. In a small bowl, combine almonds and goat cheese. Divide into 12 portions and set aside.

4. Stuff 1 wedge of sausage and 1 portion of goat cheese mixture into each date. Cheese mixture should be mounded outside the slit. Repeat process until all dates are stuffed.

5. Sprinkle with parsley.

Variation: Omit the sausage and use the cheese mixture only, or stuff the dates with whole almonds and add plain goat cheese.

HEALTHY MORSELS

Medjool dates are loved for their large size, extreme sweetness, and chewy texture. They are nature's candy bar! You can use other date varieties in this recipe, but Medjool dates are preferred.

Mushroom Crostini

In this fall dish, simple sautéed mushrooms become meaty and earthy, making a delicious topping for crostini.

Yield:	Prep time:	Cook time:	Serving size:
1¾ cups	30 minutes	20 to 30 minutes	1 crostini

Each serving has:			
30 calories	1.5 g total fat	0 g saturated fat	1 g protein
3 g carbohydrates	0 g fiber	0 mg cholesterol	45 mg sodium

⅛ cup extra-virgin olive oil

3 TB. shallot, minced

8 oz. white button mushrooms, chopped

8 oz. baby portobello mushrooms, chopped

¼ cup white wine

3 cloves garlic, minced

1 TB. fresh thyme leaves, minced

¼ tsp. kosher salt

⅛ tsp. freshly ground black pepper

1 baguette

1. Preheat oven to 375°F.

2. Heat oil in large skillet over medium heat. Add shallot and cook for 2 to 3 minutes.

3. Add mushrooms, wine, garlic, thyme, salt, and pepper. Mushrooms will give off liquid as they cook. Cook until all liquid has evaporated, approximately 10 minutes.

4. While mushrooms are cooking, slice baguette diagonally into ½-inch slices. Place baguette slices on a shallow baking sheet and toast in the oven for 4 to 5 minutes or until golden brown.

5. Spoon mushroom mixture evenly onto toasted baguette slices and serve.

Variation: For added flavor, brush bread slices with olive oil (approximately 2 tablespoons) before toasting. Rub toasted bread with raw garlic after removing from the oven.

Lemon Cannellini Spread

Lemon zest adds a refreshing zing to this summery bean spread.

Yield:	Prep time:	Cook time:	Serving size:
2 cups	10 minutes	None	¼ cup

Each serving has:			
60 calories	2 g total fat	0 g saturated fat	3 g protein
9 g carbohydrates	3 g fiber	0 mg cholesterol	140 mg sodium

1 clove garlic, peeled	1 TB. extra-virgin olive oil
1 (15-oz.) can cannellini beans, drained, liquid reserved	2 tsp. ground coriander
1 TB. lemon zest	¼ tsp. fresh rosemary leaves, chopped

1. Add garlic to a food processor and pulse until finely chopped.

2. Add cannellini beans, lemon zest, olive oil, coriander, and rosemary.

3. Purée mixture, adding reserved liquid until mixture is creamy. Use a spatula to scrape down the sides of the bowl.

4. Use as a spread on a sliced baguette or as a sandwich spread.

Variation: You can use any white bean with this recipe. Also try substituting tarragon for the rosemary.

Hummus

Savory and creamy, hummus is a great dip or sandwich spread for springtime.

Yield:	Prep time:	Cook time:	Serving size:
3½ cups	10 minutes	None	¼ cup

Each serving has:			
80 calories	4 g total fat	0 g saturated fat	3 g protein
9 g carbohydrates	2 g fiber	0 mg cholesterol	200 mg sodium

2 cloves garlic, peeled

2 (15-oz.) cans garbanzo beans, drained, liquid reserved

2 TB. fresh lemon juice

2 TB. extra-virgin olive oil

2 TB. tahini

4 tsp. ground coriander

2 tsp. cumin

½ tsp. kosher salt

⅛ tsp. freshly ground black pepper

1. Add garlic cloves to food processor. Pulse until finely chopped.

2. Add garbanzo beans, lemon juice, olive oil, tahini, coriander, cumin, salt, and pepper.

3. Purée mixture, adding reserved liquid until mixture is creamy. Use a spatula to scrape down the sides of the bowl.

Variation: Add 2 jarred roasted red peppers for a smoky flavor, or try a handful of fresh cilantro and lemon zest.

GOOD TO KNOW

Tahini is made from sesame seeds that are ground to a paste and is the consistency of peanut butter. When you buy tahini, stir it vigorously to incorporate the oil that has risen to the top.

Eggplant Rolls

Grilling gives eggplant a wonderful, smoky flavor and beautiful grill marks. It is the perfect fall dish.

Yield:	Prep time:	Cook time:	Serving size:
10 rolls	15 minutes	5 to 7 minutes	1 eggplant roll

Each serving has:			
60 calories	4.5 g total fat	1.5 g saturated fat	2 g protein
4 g carbohydrates	2 g fiber	10 mg cholesterol	190 mg sodium

⅛ cup extra-virgin olive oil

2 TB. Italian seasoning

1 tsp. dried mint leaves

½ tsp. kosher salt

⅛ tsp. freshly ground black pepper

1 medium eggplant

1 (3-oz.) block feta cheese

1. In a small bowl, combine olive oil, Italian seasoning, mint, salt, and pepper.

2. Cut eggplant lengthwise into ⅛-inch slices.

3. Brush both sides of eggplant slices with olive oil mixture.

4. On an outdoor grill or stovetop grill pan over medium heat, grill eggplant 5 to 7 minutes, turning halfway through cooking. Eggplant should be lightly browned and soft.

5. While eggplant is cooking, slice feta into ¼-inch slices. Cut each slice in half lengthwise.

6. Place 1 slice of eggplant on work surface. Place 1 piece of feta at one end of eggplant slice and roll up. Continue with remaining eggplant and feta.

7. Serve at room temperature.

Variation: Use ricotta cheese instead of feta, mixing the Italian seasoning, mint, salt, and pepper into the ricotta, or try brushing the eggplant with plain olive oil and sprinkle only with salt and pepper before grilling.

Baked Vegetable Omelet

Jump into spring with eggs, vegetables, and cheese—a savory delight any time of the day or night.

Yield:	Prep time:	Cook time:	Serving size:
9 servings	15 minutes	40 minutes	1 square
Each serving has:			
160 calories	10 g total fat	4 g saturated fat	12 g protein
5 g carbohydrates	1 g fiber	245 mg cholesterol	250 mg sodium

1 TB. extra-virgin olive oil

10 large eggs

¼ cup asparagus, thinly sliced

¼ cup red onion, finely chopped

½ cup sun-dried tomatoes, packed in oil

1 cup fresh baby spinach

¼ cup red bell pepper, cored and finely chopped

1 cup sliced mushrooms

12 oz. part-skim ricotta cheese, drained

¼ tsp. kosher salt

⅛ tsp. freshly ground black pepper

1 TB. finely chopped fresh parsley

1. Preheat oven to 350°F.

2. Coat a 9×9 pan with olive oil. Be sure to coat sides well.

3. In a large mixing bowl, add eggs and beat well.

4. In a separate large mixing bowl, add asparagus, onion, tomatoes, spinach, bell pepper, mushrooms, ricotta, salt, and pepper. Mix well.

5. Pour beaten eggs over vegetable mixture and mix well.

6. Transfer mixture to the prepared pan and bake for approximately 40 minutes or until set in the center.

7. Remove from oven and run a paring knife around the edges of the pan. Cut into 9 portions.

8. Garnish each serving with a pinch of parsley. Serve warm or at room temperature.

Variation: Roast the vegetables for a sweeter, more intense vegetable flavor. Let cool before adding to the egg mixture.

TO YOUR HEALTH

The Italian frittata is the inspiration for this dish. A frittata is cooked in a skillet on the stove over very low heat and finished in the oven under the broiler. This is a simpler version but just as delicious.

Crab Cakes

Crab cakes are always a hit in the summer months. Serve as a main course or as an appetizer.

Yield:	Prep time:	Cook time:	Serving size:
12 patties	15 minutes	15 minutes	1 patty

Each serving has:			
100 calories	4 g total fat	1 g saturated fat	9 g protein
8 g carbohydrates	0 g fiber	50 mg cholesterol	340 mg sodium

1 large egg, lightly beaten

1 TB. Dijon mustard

1 TB. light mayonnaise

2 TB. finely chopped fresh parsley

2 TB. red onion, finely diced

2 TB. red bell pepper, finely diced

1 TB. Old Bay Seasoning

1 lb. lump crabmeat

1 cup Italian-style breadcrumbs

2 TB. extra-virgin olive oil

1. Preheat oven to 400°F.

2. In a large mixing bowl, combine egg, mustard, mayonnaise, parsley, onion, bell pepper, and Old Bay Seasoning. Mix well.

3. Gently add crabmeat and breadcrumbs, taking care not to break up crabmeat.

4. Using ¼ cup crab mixture, form 1-inch thick patties. Continue until 12 patties are formed. Set aside.

5. In a large nonstick skillet over medium heat, add 1 tablespoon olive oil. When olive oil is hot, add 6 patties. Cook for 1 to 2 minutes on each side or until slightly browned. You are just adding color, not cooking patties all the way through. Transfer patties to a sheet pan. Add remaining tablespoon oil and fry remaining 6 patties. Place on the sheet pan with first batch of patties.

6. Bake patties at 400°F for 5 to 10 minutes or until golden brown.

GOOD TO KNOW

Be sure to look for high-quality lump or jumbo lump crabmeat. Processed crabmeat can contain bits of shell or cartilage, so gently pick through the crab and remove any bits that you find.

Tomato Basil Bocconcini

Sweet summer tomatoes and fresh basil is a match made in culinary heaven.

Yield:	Prep time:	Cook time:	Serving size:
2 servings	10 minutes	None	½ recipe

Each serving has:			
210 calories	14 g total fat	6 g saturated fat	15 g protein
7 g carbohydrates	1 g fiber	35 mg cholesterol	610 mg sodium

4 ounces bocconcini (about 2 mozzarella balls)

2 medium tomatoes

15 large basil leaves

2 tsp. extra-virgin olive oil

Kosher salt and freshly ground black pepper to taste

1. Slice each bocconcini ball into 4 slices.

2. Core tomatoes and cut each into 4 horizontal slices.

3. On each plate, layer 1 tomato slice, 1 basil leaf, and 1 slice bocconcini. Repeat process, making 4 stacks on each plate.

4. Drizzle with olive oil. Sprinkle with a pinch of salt and black pepper.

5. Cut remaining basil leaves into fine shreds to garnish each serving.

HEALTHY MORSELS

Bocconcini are traditionally made from the milk of water buffaloes. Today, you may find them made from water buffalo's milk or a combination of water buffalo's and cow's milk, and they can be packed in whey or water. If you cannot find bocconcini in your market, you can use any type of fresh mozzarella.

Lamb Pesto Crostini

These crostini are the perfect springtime starter before a meal, or you can serve them as an entrée paired with a salad.

Yield:	Prep time:	Cook time:	Serving size:
40 crostini	20 minutes	20 minutes	1 crostini
Each serving has:			
150 calories	6 g total fat	2 g saturated fat	7 g protein
18 g carbohydrates	1 g fiber	10 mg cholesterol	240 mg sodium

1 baguette	⅛ tsp. freshly ground black pepper
1½ lb. lamb shoulder	3 large Roma tomatoes
1 tsp. Italian seasoning	6 TB. Pesto (see recipe earlier in chapter)
⅛ tsp. kosher salt	

1. Preheat oven to 400°F.

2. Slice baguette into ⅛-inch slices. Lay slices in a single layer on an ungreased cookie sheet. Place in oven and bake for 3 to 4 minutes per side or until lightly toasted. Let cool.

3. Season lamb on both sides with Italian seasoning, salt, and pepper. On a grill set to medium heat, cook lamb for 8 to 10 minutes per side or until it reaches an internal temperature of 145°F on a meat thermometer. Remove from grill and place on a plate; cover with foil. Let rest for 5 minutes.

4. While lamb is resting, core tomatoes and slice in half lengthwise. Slice again into half-rounds approximately ⅛-inch thick.

5. Slice lamb into ⅛-inch thick slices.

6. Spread Pesto onto crostini. Place 1 tomato slice on each and top with lamb slice. Repeat process until all crostini are used.

Variation: Serve some crostini with lamb and some without—the crostini are delicious with just the pesto and tomato.

HEALTHY MORSELS

Crostini means "little toasts" and they are sometimes brushed with olive oil. Bruschetta is similar—it is toasted or grilled bread that has been brushed with olive oil and rubbed with garlic.

Lemon Minted Melon

Nice, cold melon is so refreshing in the summertime. Try it with the sweet mint sauce for an extra-special twist.

Yield:	Prep time:	Cook time:	Serving size:
4 servings	5 minutes	5 minutes	¼ melon with 1 tablespoon syrup

Each serving has:			
120 calories	0 g total fat	0 g saturated fat	1 g protein
29 g carbohydrates	1 g fiber	0 mg cholesterol	25 mg sodium

1 medium cantaloupe	1 TB. fresh mint, finely chopped
⅓ cup sugar	1 tsp. lemon zest
¼ cup water	

1. Cut cantaloupe in half and remove seeds. Slice into 12 wedges and remove peel.

2. In a small saucepan, combine sugar, water, mint, and lemon zest. Cook over medium-high heat 5 minutes or until sugar has dissolved. Let cool.

3. Drizzle 1 tablespoon syrup over 3 wedges of melon. Garnish with additional mint leaves.

Variation: Try this with any variety of melon, including honeydew, crenshaw, or canary.

TO YOUR HEALTH

To choose a ripe cantaloupe, look for a melon that is heavy for its size. The blossom end should give slightly when pressed and give off a hint of the sweet cantaloupe aroma.

Onion Apple Marmalade

When onions are caramelized as they are in this fall recipe, they become sweet and delicious.

Yield:	Prep time:	Cook time:	Serving size:
1½ cups	5 minutes	20 minutes	2 tablespoons

Each serving has:			
20 calories	0.5 g total fat	0 g saturated fat	0 g protein
4 g carbohydrates	0 g fiber	0 mg cholesterol	40 mg sodium

1 TB. extra-virgin olive oil	½ tsp. kosher salt
3 cups white onion, diced	2 TB. sugar
1 cup red delicious apple, finely diced	1 TB. apple cider vinegar
	1 TB. water

1. Heat olive oil in a large nonstick skillet over medium heat. Add onions, apple, and salt. Cook for 10 minutes, stirring occasionally.

2. Add sugar, vinegar, and water. Cook for 15 to 20 more minutes, stirring occasionally, until onions are golden brown.

3. Use as a topping for crostini or pizza, as a sandwich spread, or on grilled chicken or pork.

Parmesan Pepper Crisps

These savory cheese crisps can be served with appetizers, a salad, or a bowl of soup on a cold winter day.

Yield:	Prep time:	Cook time:	Serving size:
20 crisps	10 minutes	15 minutes	1 crisp

Each serving has:			
70 calories	2.5 g total fat	1 g saturated fat	3 g protein
10 g carbohydrates	0 g fiber	5 mg cholesterol	105 mg sodium

1 TB. extra-virgin olive oil	1 cup Parmesan cheese, shredded
2 cups all-purpose flour, plus additional flour for rolling out dough	¼ tsp. kosher salt
	1 tsp. freshly ground black pepper
	¾ cup warm water

1. Preheat oven to 400°F. Coat a sheet pan with olive oil.

2. In a large mixing bowl, combine flour, cheese, salt, and pepper. Mix well.

3. Add water and mix until dough forms a ball. Turn out onto a floured surface. Knead gently for 2 to 3 minutes.

4. Sprinkle top of dough with flour and roll out into a 12×12 square that is ⅛-inch thick.

5. Using a pizza cutter or sharp knife, cut dough into ¼-inch strips. Transfer to prepared sheet pan.

6. Cook on top rack of the oven for 12 to 15 minutes or until slightly golden.

Variation: Rosemary would be a great addition to the cheese crisps. Add 1 teaspoon chopped fresh rosemary to the flour, cheese, salt, and pepper mixture.

HEALTHY MORSELS

Fresh Parmesan cheese has so much more flavor than the preshredded varieties. Buy a wedge of fresh Parmesan and be rewarded with great flavor.

Smoked Salmon Bites

Cool, crunchy cucumber is used as the base for flavorful smoked salmon. This makes a great summer dish.

Yield:	Prep time:	Cook time:	Serving size:
12 salmon bites	15 minutes	None	1 salmon bite

Each serving has:			
80 calories	6 g total fat	1.5 g saturated fat	5 g protein
1 g carbohydrates	0 g fiber	15 mg cholesterol	125 mg sodium

2 TB. extra-virgin olive oil

2 tsp. fresh lemon juice

$\frac{1}{8}$ tsp. freshly ground black pepper

$\frac{1}{8}$ tsp. kosher salt

1 clove garlic, finely minced

1 TB. red onion, finely chopped

1 cucumber

2 TB. crumbled feta

2 TB. red bell pepper, finely chopped

1 TB. finely chopped Italian flat-leaf parsley

1 tsp. fresh basil, finely chopped

$\frac{1}{3}$ lb. smoked salmon

1. In a small mixing bowl, combine olive oil, lemon juice, pepper, salt, garlic, and onion. Mix well.

2. Cut cucumber into 12 $\frac{1}{8}$-inch rounds and set aside. With remaining cucumber, peel, seed, and dice enough for $\frac{1}{4}$ cup.

3. Add feta, diced cucumber, bell pepper, parsley, and basil to olive oil mixture. Stir to coat.

4. Cut salmon into 12 pieces.

5. Place one piece of salmon on each cucumber slice. Top with a teaspoon of vegetable mixture. Repeat process until you have 12 portions.

Variation: Instead of cucumbers, use a toasted slice of baguette or serve on an endive leaf.

TO YOUR HEALTH

There are two types of smoked salmon, cold-smoked and hot-smoked. Either type can be used in this recipe. You may see cold-smoked salmon labeled as Nova or Lox and is usually sold in very thin slices. Hot-smoked salmon is sold in large pieces and is flaky like a piece of cooked fish.

Scrumptious Soups and Salads

In This Chapter

- Soup basics
- Creating new flavors
- Salads—more than just leafy greens
- Delicious recipes

Soup has long been considered a meal throughout history and throughout the Mediterranean, and is an integral part of our lives, providing warmth, nourishment, and comfort. The basis of most Mediterranean soups is high-quality chicken, beef, or vegetable broth. You can purchase low-sodium broths or make your own, as this will allow you to control the sodium level. Most soups freeze well and make great meals, either as a satisfying dinner or a nutritious lunch at home or at the office.

Salads are another popular tradition of the Mediterranean. They can be so much more than just mixed greens. Combining fruits, vegetables, beans, and nuts with greens can make a salad that's beautiful for your eyes and delicious for your taste buds—not to mention a complete meal. From a simple cucumber salad to a more filling shrimp and melon salad, they allow great versatility and provide loads of nutrition. What you top your salad with should be just as healthy and light as the ingredients in the salad. Make your own dressing with ingredients such as extra-virgin olive oil, vinegar, mustard, shallots, herbs, and spices, and your salad will pop with flavor.

The tantalizing recipes in this chapter span all of the seasons and use fresh, seasonal ingredients. Use the recipes in season or whenever you like!

Tomato Basil Soup

Get the flavor of summer tomatoes in the winter when they aren't in season with high-quality canned tomatoes, used here in a soup that can be made anytime.

Yield:	Prep time:	Cook time:	Serving size:
4 cups	15 minutes	30 minutes	1 cup

Each serving has:			
140 calories	7 g total fat	1 g saturated fat	2 g protein
17 g carbohydrates	5 g fiber	0 mg cholesterol	350 mg sodium

2 TB. extra-virgin olive oil	1 tsp. sugar
1 cup white onion, diced	2 (14.5-oz.) cans diced tomatoes, no salt added
2 ribs celery, chopped	½ tsp. kosher salt
1 TB. garlic, minced	⅛ tsp. freshly ground black pepper
1 TB. dried basil	

1. In a large pot over medium heat, add 1 tablespoon olive oil. When heated, cook onions, celery, and garlic for 5 minutes.

2. Add basil, sugar, tomatoes with juice, salt, and pepper.

3. Bring to a boil and reduce heat to low. Simmer for 20 minutes.

4. Add remaining 1 tablespoon olive oil. Purée in blender in batches, or use an immersion blender to purée in the pot.

5. Once puréed, cook for an additional 10 minutes.

TO YOUR HEALTH

Salt is added to this recipe even though no-salt-added canned tomatoes are called for. Processed foods can contain large amounts of sodium. Purchase no-salt-added products and add the salt yourself to help control the amount of sodium in your diet.

Lemon Lentil Soup

The hint of lemon and tangy yogurt adds a wonderful flavor dimension to the simple and humble winter lentil soup.

Yield:	Prep time:	Cook time:	Serving size:
10 cups	15 minutes	30 minutes	1 cup soup with 2 tablespoons yogurt

Each serving has:			
190 calories	3 g total fat	0.5 g saturated fat	13 g protein
30 g carbohydrates	7 g fiber	0 mg cholesterol	150 mg sodium

1 TB. extra-virgin olive oil	1 tsp. dried oregano leaves
1 cup onion, diced	¼ tsp. freshly ground black pepper
½ cup celery, sliced ¼-inch thick	1 TB. ground coriander
½ cup carrots, sliced ¼-inch thick	Zest of one lemon
8 cups vegetable broth	1 cup kale, shredded
2 cups red lentils	1¼ cups plain Greek yogurt
2 dried bay leaves	Sprigs of fresh parsley
1 garlic clove, minced	

1. Heat a large stockpot over medium heat, add olive oil. When heated, add onion, celery, and carrots. Cook for 5 minutes, stirring occasionally.

2. Add vegetable broth, lentils, bay leaves, garlic, oregano, pepper, and coriander. Stir to combine. Heat to medium-high and bring soup to a boil. Reduce heat to low and simmer for 20 minutes, stirring occasionally.

3. Stir in lemon zest and kale. Cook for 5 minutes until kale is wilted.

4. Remove and discard bay leaves.

5. Serve 1 cup of soup with 2 tablespoons of yogurt. Garnish with parsley sprigs.

Variation: Add a tablespoon of finely diced pancetta or bacon along with the vegetables in step 1.

HEALTHY MORSELS

Lemon juice and lemon zest are a great way to decrease sodium in soups. It really perks up the flavor!

Butternut Squash Soup

Sweet butternut squash is delicious and creamy. It's comfort in a cup on a chilly winter night.

Yield:	Prep time:	Cook time:	Serving size:
6 cups	15 minutes	40 minutes	1 cup

Each serving has:			
190 calories	3.5 g total fat	0.5 g saturated fat	6 g protein
39 g carbohydrates	6 g fiber	0 mg cholesterol	230 mg sodium

2 medium butternut squash (about 3 lb.)	1 garlic clove, minced
1 TB. extra-virgin olive oil	$\frac{1}{2}$ tsp. kosher salt
1 cup white onion, diced	$\frac{1}{8}$ tsp. freshly ground black pepper
1 tsp. Italian seasoning	1 TB. honey
4 cups low-sodium chicken broth	$1\frac{1}{2}$ tsp. fresh ginger, peeled, finely grated

1. Preheat oven to 400°F.

2. Cut squash in half lengthwise and remove seeds. Place on a baking sheet cut side down. Bake for 30 to 45 minutes or until a knife is easily inserted.

3. When squash is cool enough to handle, use a spoon to remove flesh from skin and set aside.

4. In a large pot over medium heat, add olive oil and heat until shimmering. Add onions and cook for 5 to 7 minutes, stirring occasionally. Add Italian seasoning and stir to combine.

5. To the pot, add squash, 3 cups chicken broth, garlic, salt, pepper, honey, and ginger. Cook over low heat for 20 minutes.

6. Purée half mixture with an immersion stick blender, or transfer half to a food processor or blender and purée. Do not fill the blender more than $\frac{1}{2}$ full in each batch as hot liquids will expand when blended. Remove the center of the blender lid to allow steam to escape. Place a kitchen towel over the top. Purée 1 minute until smooth. Transfer to a large bowl and repeat with remaining soup.

7. Pour puréed soup back into pot. Add remaining 1 cup chicken broth. Cook for an additional 10 minutes.

Vegetable Orzo Soup

A real springtime soup, and one that's easy to make.

Yield:	Prep time:	Cook time:	Serving size:
5 cups	20 minutes	30 minutes	1 cup

Each serving has:			
120 calories	4 g total fat	0 g saturated fat	6 g protein
16 g carbohydrates	2 g fiber	0 mg cholesterol	260 mg sodium

1 TB. extra-virgin olive oil	1 cup mushrooms, sliced
¼ cup celery, chopped	1 clove garlic, finely minced
½ cup onion, diced	½ cup *orzo*
¼ cup carrots, sliced	1 tsp. Italian seasoning
1 (14.5-oz.) can diced tomatoes, no salt added	½ tsp. kosher salt
4 cups low-sodium chicken broth	¼ tsp. freshly ground black pepper
1 cup zucchini, chopped	Sprigs of fresh parsley

1. In a large stockpot over medium heat, add olive oil. When heated, add celery, onion, and carrots. Cook for 5 minutes, stirring occasionally.

2. Add tomatoes with liquid, chicken broth, zucchini, mushrooms, garlic, orzo, Italian seasoning, salt, and pepper. Increase heat slightly and bring to a gentle boil. Cook for 25 minutes, stirring occasionally.

3. Garnish with parsley sprigs.

Variation: Add 1 link cooked spicy Italian sausage to the soup. Cut into slices and add along with the tomatoes.

DEFINITION

Orzo is small, rice-shaped pasta. It looks like a large grain of rice but is made from the same semolina flour as any pasta. It is widely available in the pasta aisle of most supermarkets.

Split Pea Soup

Sweet and smoky comfort in a bowl, this soup is perfect for wintertime.

Yield:	Prep time:	Cook time:	Serving size:
8 cups	15 minutes	45 minutes	1 cup

Each serving has:			
260 calories	4.5 g total fat	1 g saturated fat	18 g protein
37 g carbohydrates	15 g fiber	20 mg cholesterol	240 mg sodium

1 TB. extra-virgin olive oil	2 tsp. ground coriander
1 cup yellow onion, diced	1 tsp. dried oregano
½ cup celery, diced	¼ tsp. freshly ground black pepper
½ cup carrots, diced	6 cups low-sodium chicken stock
1 smoked ham hock	16 oz. dried split peas
2 cloves garlic, minced	8 fresh chives, minced

1. In a large stockpot over medium heat, add olive oil. When heated, add onion, celery, and carrots. Cook for 5 minutes.

2. Add ham hock, garlic, coriander, oregano, and pepper. Stir together and cook for 1 minute.

3. Increase the heat slightly and add chicken broth and peas. Bring to a boil, and then cover and reduce heat to a simmer. Cook for 40 to 50 minutes or until peas are tender.

4. Remove the ham hock, or if desired, shred meat and add back to the soup after it has been blended.

5. Purée half mixture with an immersion stick blender, or transfer half to a food processor or blender and purée.

6. Garnish with fresh chives.

Variation: Add crispy pancetta or bacon as a garnish.

Gazpacho

This cold soup is bright-tasting with ripe summer tomatoes and is refreshing on a hot summer day.

Yield:	Prep time:	Cook time:	Serving size:
3 cups	20 minutes	5 minutes	¾ cup

Each serving has:			
60 calories	4 g total fat	0.5 g saturated fat	2 g protein
7 g carbohydrates	2 g fiber	0 mg cholesterol	260 mg sodium

8 large tomatoes	1 TB. fresh lemon juice
½ cup celery, diced	1 tsp. lemon zest
½ cup cucumber, peeled, seeded, and diced	½ tsp. kosher salt
	⅛ tsp. freshly ground black pepper
4 scallions, sliced, white parts only	1 TB. minced fresh parsley
1 clove garlic, minced	1 TB. extra-virgin olive oil

1. In medium stockpot, bring 3 quarts of water to a boil.

2. In a large mixing bowl, add 2 cups of ice and fill with cold water.

3. Cut a small *X* into the bottom of each tomato. Place 4 tomatoes into boiling water and cook 30 seconds. Remove with a slotted spoon or tongs and place immediately into ice water. Repeat with remaining tomatoes.

4. Peel tomatoes starting at the *X*. Once peeled, roughly chop and transfer to a food processor.

5. Add celery, cucumber, scallions, garlic, lemon juice, lemon zest, salt, pepper, parsley, and olive oil to the food processor. Pulse 3 to 4 times to roughly chop ingredients. Remove half mixture and place in a large bowl.

6. With food processor, purée the remaining mixture. Transfer puréed ingredients to the large bowl and mix with roughly chopped ingredients.

7. Refrigerate at least 1 hour to meld the flavors. Garnish with additional chopped cucumber and a drizzle of extra-virgin olive oil.

Mixed Bean Soup

Hearty, savory, and satisfying, this fall bean soup can stand alone as a meal.

Yield:	Prep time:	Cook time:	Serving size:
6 cups	15 minutes	2½ hours	1 cup

Each serving has:			
200 calories	10 g total fat	3 g saturated fat	8 g protein
20 g carbohydrates	6 g fiber	10 mg cholesterol	910 mg sodium

1 cup dry pinto or cranberry beans	½ cup carrots, diced
1 cup dry white beans	8 cups low-sodium chicken broth
1 TB. extra-virgin olive oil	1 TB. Italian seasoning
1 cup white onion, diced	⅛ tsp. freshly ground black pepper
½ cup celery, diced	1 smoked ham hock

1. Pick through dried beans and remove any stones.

2. In a large bowl, add beans. Cover with enough cold water so they will remain covered as they double in size. Soak beans overnight. Remove any bad-looking beans. Drain and rinse.

3. In a medium stockpot over medium heat, add oil. When heated, add onion, celery, and carrots. Sauté for 5 minutes.

4. Add chicken broth, beans, Italian seasoning, pepper, and ham hock. Increase heat to high.

5. Bring to a rolling boil, then lower to medium heat. Cook for 2½ to 3 hours or until beans are tender.

6. Remove the ham hock, or if desired, shred meat and add back to the beans.

Variation: Any bean can be used with this recipe, mixing and matching as many types of beans as you like. Just keep the total at 2 cups.

HEALTHY MORSELS

Cranberry beans have a creamy texture and are cream colored with deep red or cranberry-colored markings. As pretty as they are when dried, they do not keep the red markings when cooked.

Marinated Artichoke Salad

The flavors of an antipasto platter are combined here for a quick and delicious wintertime salad.

Yield:	Prep time:	Cook time:	Serving size:
3 cups	15 minutes	None	½ cup

Each serving has:			
90 calories	5 g total fat	1.5 g saturated fat	3 g protein
9 g carbohydrates	3 g fiber	5 mg cholesterol	600 mg sodium

⅓ cup canned artichoke hearts in water, drained

¼ cup Kalamata olives, pitted and chopped

⅓ cup jarred roasted red peppers, chopped

¼ cup feta cheese, crumbled

2 TB. red onion, finely chopped

1 TB. extra-virgin olive oil

1 TB. balsamic vinegar

1 clove garlic, finely minced

1 TB. finely chopped fresh parsley

⅛ tsp. kosher salt

⅛ tsp. freshly ground black pepper

1. In a large mixing bowl, combine artichoke hearts, Kalamata olives, red peppers, feta cheese, onion, olive oil, vinegar, garlic, parsley, salt, and pepper. Mix well.

2. Cover and refrigerate for at least 30 minutes to allow flavors to meld.

3. Serve the recipe as a small salad or as a side to go along with a variety of appetizers.

Variation: Add 2 ounces each of sliced cheese and salami and serve on a bed of mixed greens.

Roasted Beet Salad

Fall is a great time for roasting beets, which brings out their delicious sweet and earthy flavor that even beet-haters will love.

Yield:	Prep time:	Cook time:	Serving size:
About 4 cups	30 minutes	2 hours	1 cup

Each serving has:			
190 calories	15 g total fat	4 g saturated fat	4 g protein
10 g carbohydrates	2 g fiber	15 mg cholesterol	270 mg sodium

2 large beets

3 TB. extra-virgin olive oil

1 TB. shallot, finely chopped

1 clove garlic, minced

1 TB. apple cider vinegar

¼ tsp. Dijon mustard

1½ tsp. fresh mint leaves, finely chopped

2 tsp. honey

½ tsp. lemon zest

⅛ tsp. kosher salt

⅛ tsp. freshly ground black pepper

1 cup romaine lettuce, shredded

2 oz. feta cheese

2 TB. pistachios (purchased pre-roasted and salted), chopped

1. Preheat oven to 400°F.

2. Remove any greens from beets. Wrap each beet in aluminum foil. Bake for 1 hour or until knife-tender. Remove from oven and cool.

3. When beets are completely cool, use a paring knife to peel. Cut beets into 1-inch cubes and place in medium bowl.

4. In a small bowl, make the dressing by combining olive oil, shallot, garlic, apple cider vinegar, mustard, mint, honey, lemon zest, salt, and pepper.

5. Add 2 tablespoons dressing to cubed beets.

6. Toss 1 tablespoon dressing with shredded lettuce.

7. Arrange salad on plates using ¼ cup lettuce, approximately 1 cup of beets, and ½ oz. feta cheese. Top with ½ tablespoon pistachios.

TO YOUR HEALTH

Don't throw away those beet greens—they are delicious! You can use beet greens as you would other dark leafy greens. Wash and tear into 2- to 3-inch pieces and sauté in olive oil and garlic until wilted.

Golden Couscous Salad

The sweetness of the golden raisins complements the curry essence of the couscous. It is a great summer side dish with grilled lamb or chicken.

Yield:	Prep time:	Cook time:	Serving size:
10 cups	20 minutes	15 minutes	½ cup
Each serving has:			
80 calories	2.5 g total fat	0 g saturated fat	2 g protein
12 g carbohydrates	1 g fiber	0 mg cholesterol	50 mg sodium

2 TB. extra-virgin olive oil

8 oz. Israeli couscous

2 cups warm water

⅓ cup golden raisins

½ tsp. curry powder

1 clove garlic, finely minced

½ cup red bell pepper, cored and finely chopped

½ cup celery, finely diced

4 scallions, finely minced

1 tsp. orange zest

½ tsp. kosher salt

⅛ tsp. freshly ground black pepper

¼ cup pine nuts, toasted

1. In a small pot over medium heat, add tablespoon olive oil. When heated, add couscous. Cook until slightly toasted, about 5 minutes, stirring occasionally.

2. To the pot, add 2 cups warm water, raisins, and curry powder and mix well. Bring to a boil, then reduce heat to a simmer and cover. Simmer 15 minutes or until all liquid is absorbed. Remove from heat. Transfer to a large mixing bowl and cool to room temperature.

3. In a small skillet over medium heat, toast pine nuts for 5 to 6 minutes until lightly browned.

4. When couscous has cooled, add garlic, bell pepper, celery, scallions, orange zest, remaining 1 tablespoon olive oil, salt, pepper, and pine nuts. Mix well. Refrigerate at least 30 minutes to meld the flavors.

 HEALTHY MORSELS

Israeli couscous is larger than the couscous you may be familiar with. Israeli couscous is white and is the size of a small pea. You can also use whole-grain couscous to up your fiber intake.

Tuna Salad with Capers and Potatoes

This light, refreshing version of tuna salad is perfect for warmer months. It's very different than the mayonnaise-based version many of us are familiar with.

Yield:	Prep time:	Cook time:	Serving size:
4 servings	15 minutes	15 minutes	⅓ cup tuna mixture, 2 ounces potato, and 1 cup lettuce

Each serving has:			
200 calories	10 g total fat	1.5 g saturated fat	13 g protein
15 g carbohydrates	3 g fiber	15 mg cholesterol	510 mg sodium

8 oz. new potatoes	1 TB. red onion, minced
4 TB. balsamic vinaigrette	2 TB. *capers*
10 cherry tomatoes, halved	1 (6-oz.) can solid albacore tuna, in spring water, drained
10 Kalamata olives, pitted and halved	4 cups mixed lettuce greens

1. In a medium pot over medium-high heat, boil potatoes for 15 minutes or until knife-tender. Remove from water and cool to room temperature.

2. When potatoes have cooled, slice ¼-inch thick. In a small mixing bowl, gently mix 1 tablespoon balsamic vinaigrette with potatoes.

3. In a separate mixing bowl, combine tomatoes, olives, onion, capers, tuna, and 2 tablespoons of balsamic vinaigrette. Gently mix.

4. In a separate mixing bowl, toss lettuce greens with remaining 1 tablespoon balsamic vinaigrette, coating well.

5. To serve, place 1 cup of lettuce greens on each of 4 plates. Top evenly with sliced potato and ⅓ cup tuna mixture.

DEFINITION

Capers are the immature buds plucked from a small caper bush that is native to the Mediterranean and Middle East. The buds are picked and then dried and pickled.

Fennel and Apple Salad

The slight licorice flavor of fennel combines with sweet apples for this bright, refreshing winter salad.

Yield:	Prep time:	Cook time:	Serving size:
4 cups	20 minutes	None	1 cup

Each serving has:			
210 calories	14 g total fat	2 g saturated fat	2 g protein
23 g carbohydrates	6 g fiber	0 mg cholesterol	170 mg sodium

¼ cup extra-virgin olive oil	⅛ tsp. freshly ground black pepper
1 clove garlic, finely minced	4 scallions
1 TB. fresh lemon juice	2 medium red delicious apples
1 TB. lemon zest	1 fennel bulb
¼ tsp. kosher salt	1 cup baby spinach

1. In a large mixing bowl, combine olive oil, garlic, lemon juice, lemon zest, salt, and pepper.

2. Cut scallions, separating the white parts from the green tops. Finely mince the white parts and add to mixing bowl. Cut the green tops diagonally into ⅛-inch thick slices and add to the mixing bowl. Mix well.

3. Slice apples into ⅛-inch thick slices. Cut across the slices into ⅛-inch thick sticks. Immediately toss the apple into the olive oil mixture to prevent browning, mixing well after each addition. There is no need to core the apples as you slice from the outer edges toward the core. You can discard the middle that contains the core.

4. Remove green stalks and fronds from fennel bulb. Slice fennel bulb in half through the center of the root. Cut out hard triangular core and discard. Slice fennel into thin slices, using a mandolin slicer if you have one. Add to mixing bowl and toss well.

5. Add spinach to the mixing bowl. Toss to coat.

Variation: Add ½ cup pomegranate seeds or 1 cup grapes, cut in half.

Shrimp and Melon Salad

Shrimp and sweet summer melon are a great pairing in this refreshing summer salad.

Yield:	Prep time:	Cook time:	Serving size:
2 servings	15 minutes	None	½ recipe

Each serving has:			
250 calories	22 g total fat	3 g saturated fat	8 g protein
9 g carbohydrates	4 g fiber	55 mg cholesterol	200 mg sodium

2 cups red leaf lettuce, torn into bite-size pieces

⅓ cup cantaloupe, cut into ½-inch cubes

1 scallion, white and green parts, finely chopped

½ Hass avocado, diced

½ lb. (26 to 30 count, about 14) cooked shrimp, tails left on

2 TB. balsamic vinaigrette

1 TB. fresh basil, finely chopped

1. Place 1 cup of lettuce on each plate.

2. Divide cantaloupe, scallion, and avocado evenly between each plate.

3. Top each plate with 7 shrimp. Stand shrimp in center of salad mixture with tails pointing up.

4. Top each serving with 1 tablespoon balsamic vinaigrette. Garnish with ½ teaspoon basil.

Minted Cucumber Salad

The crunch of the cool cucumber and the fresh minty flavor in this salad will cool you down on a hot summer's day.

Yield:	Prep time:	Cook time:	Serving size:
1 cup	10 minutes	None	½ cup

Each serving has:			
70 calories	7 g total fat	1 g saturated fat	1 g protein
2 g carbohydrates	1 g fiber	0 mg cholesterol	120 mg sodium

1 TB. extra-virgin olive oil

⅛ tsp. kosher salt

⅛ tsp. freshly ground black pepper

1 TB. red onion, finely minced

1 TB. fresh mint leaves, finely chopped

1 English cucumber or regular cucumber

1. In a medium mixing bowl, combine olive oil, salt, pepper, onion, and mint. Mix well.

2. Peel cucumber. Slice in half lengthwise. Scoop out the seeds with a small spoon. Now slice cucumber into ⅛-inch slices. Add to olive oil mixture. Stir to combine.

3. Let mixture rest 20 minutes and serve at room temperature.

Variation: Use basil instead of mint and serve on a bed of lettuce greens. Make it a meal by adding ½ cup cooked shrimp.

Spinach, Orange, and Feta Salad

Spinach used raw as a salad green has a completely different flavor and texture than cooked spinach, as you will discover in this favorite summer salad.

Yield:	Prep time:	Cook time:	Serving size:
4 cups	20 minutes	None	2 cups

Each serving has:			
340 calories	23 g total fat	6 g saturated fat	8 g protein
31 g carbohydrates	7 g fiber	25 mg cholesterol	390 mg sodium

2 medium oranges

3 TB. extra-virgin olive oil

1 TB. white balsamic vinegar

¼ tsp. Dijon mustard

1 tsp. Italian seasoning

1 tsp. shallot, minced

1 TB. freshly squeezed orange juice

1 tsp. honey

2 cups packed baby spinach, washed thoroughly

2 oz. feta cheese

¼ cucumber, peeled, seeded, and diced

¼ cup chopped pecans, toasted

¼ cup red onion, sliced into rings

1. On a cutting board, cut off tops and bottoms of oranges. Place oranges cut side down on the cutting board. Cut off peel and white pith, slicing from top to bottom of each orange.

2. Holding orange over a bowl to catch any juices, cut segments out of orange, leaving the membrane between each section behind. Place orange sections in a small bowl.

3. Squeeze remaining orange membrane over bowl to catch juice.

4. In a small bowl, make dressing by combining olive oil, vinegar, mustard, Italian seasoning, shallot, orange juice, and honey. Whisk to combine.

5. In a large bowl, toss 1 tablespoon dressing with spinach.

6. Add orange slices, feta cheese, and cucumber. Toss to combine.

7. Top with toasted pecans and red onion.

8. Drizzle with extra dressing if desired.

Variation: Use toasted almonds, pine nuts, or pistachios. (See the "To Your Health" sidebar following the next recipe for directions on toasting nuts.)

Classic Mixed Greens Salad with Balsamic Vinaigrette

There should be a basic green salad recipe in every kitchen. A fresh salad can be served alongside any meal and is perfect by itself as a summertime lunch.

Yield:	Prep time:	Cook time:	Serving size:
4 servings	15 minutes	None	1¼ cups salad

Each serving has:			
190 calories	19 g total fat	2.5 g saturated fat	2 g protein
7 g carbohydrates	2 g fiber	0 mg cholesterol	160 mg sodium

4 cups mixed salad greens	¼ tsp. Italian seasoning
½ cup radishes, sliced	¼ tsp. Dijon mustard
½ cup cherry tomatoes, halved	¼ tsp. kosher salt
¼ cup carrots, shredded	⅛ tsp. freshly ground black pepper
¼ cup extra-virgin olive oil	½ tsp. sugar
1 TB. balsamic vinegar	¼ cup walnuts, toasted, coarsely chopped
1 TB. shallot, finely minced	

1. Combine salad greens, radishes, tomatoes, and carrots. Toss to combine.

2. In a small mixing bowl, combine olive oil, vinegar, shallot, Italian seasoning, mustard, salt, pepper, and sugar. Whisk well to combine.

3. Pour dressing over lettuce mixture and toss to coat.

4. Divide the salad equally among 4 plates. Garnish with toasted walnuts.

Variation: The balsamic vinaigrette works well with just about any fruits, vegetables, and meats. Keep it on hand in your kitchen and you'll be drizzling it on a multitude of recipes.

TO YOUR HEALTH

Toasting any nut brings out its full flavor. To toast nuts, place them in a single layer in a small skillet over medium heat. Cook 5 to 7 minutes, stirring occasionally until they are lightly browned. Keep an eye on them, as they can turn from brown to black quickly. You can also toast them in a preheated oven at 400°F for 5 to 7 minutes.

Tabbouleh Salad

Bulgur has a nice nutty flavor. Its tender, chewy texture balances nicely with the vegetables and herbs in this fall salad.

Yield:	Prep time:	Cook time:	Serving size:
3 cups	3 hours (includes soaking time)	None	½ cup

Each serving has:			
70 calories	2.5 g total fat	0 g saturated fat	2 g protein
11 g carbohydrates	3 g fiber	0 mg cholesterol	10 mg sodium

½ cup bulgur wheat

1 cup water

½ cup finely chopped fresh parsley

⅓ cup tomato, cored, finely diced

¼ cup scallions, thinly sliced

1 cup cucumber, peeled, seeded, and finely diced

⅓ cup fresh mint leaves, finely chopped

1 TB. extra-virgin olive oil

1 TB. fresh lemon juice

1. Place bulgur in a large bowl. Add water to cover bulgur. Let soak in refrigerator for 2½ hours or overnight. The wheat will absorb water and double in size.

2. Add parsley, tomato, scallions, cucumber, and mint to the bulgur and mix well.

3. Add olive oil and lemon juice, mix well.

Fabulous Flatbreads, Pizza, and More

In This Chapter

- New ideas for pizza toppings
- A new take on the sandwich
- Tasty recipes

Flatbreads are versatile and make a quick substitute for your traditional pizza. This type of bread has been a prominent food in many different cultures. In Persia and central Asia you would find flatbread in the form of na'an. In the Middle East you would discover pita and lavash. No matter what you call it, flatbread can be the basis for a nutrient-rich snack, lunch, or dinner, topped with just about anything your heart desires, including heart-healthy Mediterranean ingredients.

Who doesn't love a good pizza? The bonus is that pizza can actually be good for you! Making pizza at home is easy with the premade dough that is readily available in many local grocery chains. You can purchase traditional white dough, whole-wheat dough, or even flavored varieties like garlic and herb. Making pizza at home also allows you to control your toppings, which enables you to gear it toward your healthier Mediterranean style of eating.

Wraps and sandwiches don't have to be the usual meat, cheese, and mayonnaise combination. You can give them a Mediterranean flair by filling them with raw or grilled vegetables, avocados, beans, hummus, herbs, and spices. Top them with a zingy yogurt topping, olive oil, or red wine vinegar.

The tasty recipes in this chapter span all of the seasons and use fresh, seasonal ingredients. Use the recipes in season or whenever you like!

Caramelized Onion Flatbread

Almost everyone loves pizza. Try a fall Mediterranean version with sweet caramelized onions as a base.

Yield:	Prep time:	Cook time:	Serving size:
1 flatbread	10 minutes	20 minutes	¼ flatbread
Each serving has:			
160 calories	9 g total fat	3 g saturated fat	6 g protein
15 g carbohydrates	2 g fiber	15 mg cholesterol	290 mg sodium

1 TB. extra-virgin olive oil

1 large sweet onion, sliced ⅛-inch thick

1 oz. pancetta, diced

1 oz. fresh mozzarella, sliced

1 (3-oz.) flatbread

1 TB. finely chopped fresh parsley

1. Preheat oven to 400°F.

2. In a large skillet over medium heat, add oil. When heated, add onion and cook for 20 minutes, stirring occasionally, until onions are golden brown. Remove from heat.

3. In a small skillet over medium heat, cook pancetta for 10 minutes or until crisp. Remove from heat and drain on a paper towel.

4. Place flatbread on an oiled cookie sheet and spread onions over top of flatbread. Sprinkle pancetta over onions and top with sliced mozzarella. Bake for 8 to 10 minutes or until cheese is melted.

5. Garnish with parsley.

Variation: Use any type of cheese you like. Blue cheese would be great with this recipe. You can also use prosciutto, bacon, or ham instead of pancetta.

Pear, Cheese, and Balsamic Flatbread

Sweet fall pears, sharp cheese, and sweet, savory balsamic syrup balance each other beautifully.

Yield:	Prep time:	Cook time:	Serving size:
1 flatbread	10 minutes	10 minutes	¼ flatbread

Each serving has:			
140 calories	4.5 g total fat	2.5 g saturated fat	6 g protein
19 g carbohydrates	4 g fiber	10 mg cholesterol	210 mg sodium

1 (3-oz.) flatbread	1 TB. Asiago cheese, shredded
1 red pear, cored	1 TB. balsamic syrup
1½ oz. provolone cheese	

1. Preheat oven to 400°F.

2. Place flatbread on an oiled sheet pan.

3. Slice pear in half. Slice one pear half into very thin slices, less than ⅛-inch thick. Reserve other half pear for another use.

4. Top flatbread with provolone. Place sliced pears on top of provolone, with the skin side all facing the same direction.

5. Sprinkle with Asiago cheese.

6. Bake for 8 to 10 minutes or until edges are slightly golden.

7. Drizzle top of flatbread with balsamic syrup. Cut into 4 pieces.

Variation: Try different cheeses in place of the provolone such as Brie, Gorgonzola, or pecorino Romano. Garnish with 1 teaspoon fresh chopped mint or 1 tablespoon toasted walnuts.

TO YOUR HEALTH

Red pears are a different variety than their green or yellow counterparts. The red pear makes a beautiful presentation in this dish, but feel free to use any type of pear you enjoy.

Tomato Basil Pizza

Fresh, juicy summer tomatoes and sweet, aromatic basil are a perfect match. Mozzarella adds a creamy, smooth richness.

Yield:	Prep time:	Cook time:	Serving size:
1 pizza	15 minutes	10–12 minutes	⅛ pizza
Each serving has:			
160 calories	5 g total fat	1 g saturated fat	7 g protein
25 g carbohydrates	1 g fiber	5 mg cholesterol	260 mg sodium

16 oz. purchased pizza dough

1 TB. Pesto (recipe in Chapter 17)

2 large Roma tomatoes, sliced
 ¼-inch thick

3 oz. fresh mozzarella, sliced
 ¼-inch thick

1 TB. fresh basil, thinly sliced

⅛ tsp. freshly ground black pepper

1. Preheat oven according to directions on pizza dough package.

2. Place pizza dough on a well-floured surface and roll out to a 12-inch round. Transfer to an oiled sheet pan.

3. Brush pizza dough with Pesto. Layer sliced tomatoes and mozzarella over Pesto.

4. Bake for 10 minutes or until edges are slightly browned.

5. Remove from oven and top with fresh basil and pepper. Cut into 8 pieces.

Variation: Try this pizza with ⅓ cup sun-dried tomatoes instead of fresh. Or, sprinkle with 2 tablespoons toasted pine nuts.

Butternut Squash and Goat Cheese Pizza

Sweet butternut squash and tangy goat cheese pair beautifully on this wintertime pizza.

Yield:	Prep time:	Cook time:	Serving size:
1 pizza	10 minutes	18 minutes	⅛ pizza

Each serving has:			
190 calories	7 g total fat	2 g saturated fat	6 g protein
27 g carbohydrates	1 g fiber	5 mg cholesterol	290 mg sodium

16 oz. purchased pizza dough

1 TB. extra-virgin olive oil

1 cup butternut squash, peeled, seeded, and diced into ⅛-inch cubes

¼ cup onion, diced

¼ tsp. kosher salt

⅛ tsp. freshly ground black pepper

1 clove garlic, finely minced

1 tsp. fresh thyme leaves, chopped

1 TB. white wine

2 oz. goat cheese

2 TB. toasted walnuts, chopped

1 TB. finely chopped fresh parsley

1. Preheat oven according to directions on pizza dough package.

2. Place pizza dough on a well-floured surface and roll out to a 12-inch round. Transfer to an oiled sheet pan.

3. In large sauté pan over medium heat, add olive oil. When heated, add squash, onion, salt, and pepper. Cook for 8 minutes, stirring occasionally.

4. Add garlic, thyme, and white wine. Cook for 2 more minutes. Remove from heat.

5. Spread warm squash mixture evenly over pizza dough. Crumble goat cheese over squash mixture.

6. Bake for 8 to 10 minutes in the center of the oven or until the edges are slightly golden.

7. Garnish with walnuts and parsley. Cut into 8 pieces.

Variation: Try using ½ teaspoon fresh rosemary instead of the tablespoon of parsley. Gorgonzola instead of goat cheese would also be a nice substitution.

TO YOUR HEALTH

Many supermarkets sell containers of fresh butternut squash already peeled and cubed. It's a great time-saver.

Veggie Wrap

Roasting summer vegetables brings out their natural sweetness and intensifies the flavor.

Yield:	Prep time:	Cook time:	Serving size:
4 wraps	30 minutes	40 to 50 minutes	½ wrap (makes 8 servings)

Each serving has:			
250 calories	11 g total fat	3.5 g saturated fat	8 g protein
30 g carbohydrates	5 g fiber	15 mg cholesterol	590 mg sodium

1 red bell pepper

1 orange bell pepper

2 TB. extra-virgin olive oil

½ tsp. kosher salt

⅛ tsp. freshly ground black pepper

1 tsp. dried mint leaves

1 tsp. coriander

1 TB. Italian seasoning

2 medium zucchini, sliced lengthwise, ¼-inch thick

1 medium eggplant, sliced lengthwise, ¼-inch thick

1 red onion, sliced into ¼-inch rings

1 cup Hummus (recipe in Chapter 17)

4 lavash-style soft flatbreads

4 oz. feta cheese, crumbled

1 cup cucumber, grated

1. Preheat oven broiler. Cut tops and bottoms off of red and orange peppers. Slice down one side of each pepper and open. Remove ribs and seeds. Place on oiled baking sheet and press to flatten with skin side up. Place peppers 2 inches from the broiler. Broil 8 to 10 minutes or until tops of peppers are charred. Remove from oven and cover with aluminum foil to let rest.

2. Preheat oven to 400°F.

3. In a small bowl, combine olive oil, salt, pepper, mint, coriander, and Italian seasoning. Brush zucchini, eggplant, and onion on both sides with olive oil mixture.

4. Spread zucchini, eggplant, and onion in a single layer onto an oiled shallow rimmed baking sheet. Bake for 30 to 40 minutes or until tender and lightly browned.

5. While vegetables are baking, remove charred skin from peppers by peeling off the blackened skin. Use a knife tip to help scrape it away from the flesh if needed and discard. Slice the pepper into thin strips.

6. Spread ¼ cup Hummus onto each flatbread. Place ¼ of the zucchini, eggplant, peppers, and onions on each flatbread. Sprinkle 1 ounce of feta cheese over vegetables. Roll up and slice in half. Serve with grated cucumber.

Chicken Tzatziki Pita

This chicken sandwich and its cool, garlicky tzatziki sauce is a delicious summer meal in a pita.

Yield:	Prep time:	Cook time:	Serving size:
2 sandwiches	10 minutes	20 minutes	1 sandwich

Each serving has:			
320 calories	10 g total fat	5 g saturated fat	33 g protein
22 g carbohydrates	2 g fiber	75 mg cholesterol	500 mg sodium

8 oz. boneless, skinless chicken breast

1 tsp. extra-virgin olive oil

¼ tsp. Italian seasoning

¼ tsp. kosher salt

⅛ tsp. freshly ground black pepper

½ cup plain Greek yogurt

¼ cup cucumber, peeled, seeded, finely chopped

1 small clove garlic, finely minced

1 small tomato, thinly sliced

6 rings red onion thinly sliced

1 pita, cut in half to form a pocket

1 TB. finely chopped fresh parsley

1. Mix olive oil, Italian seasoning, ⅛ teaspoon salt, and pepper. Add chicken to coat.

2. Over medium heat, grill chicken for 8 to 10 minutes per side or until internal temperature of 165°F is measured on a meat thermometer in thickest part of breast. Remove from heat and let rest.

3. In a small mixing bowl, make tzatziki sauce by combining remaining ⅛ teaspoon salt, yogurt, cucumber, and garlic.

4. Slice chicken breast into ¼-inch slices. Spread a tablespoon of tzatziki sauce in each pita half. Divide chicken, tomato, and onion between two pita halves. Garnish with parsley.

Variation: Bake the chicken instead of grilling. Place the chicken on a baking sheet and bake at 375°F for about 30 minutes.

HEALTHY MORSELS

Tzatziki is a common condiment in Greece and Turkey and is served with souvlaki and gyros. It can also be used as a dip with pita wedges.

Prosciutto and Roasted Vegetable Panini

Silky smooth prosciutto has the flavor of very mild ham with just a hint of salt. Paired with summer roasted vegetables and melted cheese, it is fabulous.

Yield:	Prep time:	Cook time:	Serving size:
2 sandwiches	10 minutes	5 minutes	1 sandwich
Each serving has:			
450 calories	20 g total fat	7 g saturated fat	23 g protein
48 g carbohydrates	5 g fiber	40 mg cholesterol	1450 mg sodium

4 slices potato bread

2 tsp. extra-virgin olive oil

2 oz. provolone cheese

2 oz. prosciutto

⅔ cup roasted vegetables

1. Brush one side of each slice of bread with olive oil. Place two pieces of bread on the panini press, oiled side down.

2. Place one slice of provolone on each slice of bread. Top with 1 ounce prosciutto, and ⅓ cup roasted vegetables. Cover with remaining slices of bread, oiled side up.

3. Cook in a panini press for 3 minutes or until golden brown. If you do not have a panini press, cook in a nonstick skillet over medium heat. Cook 3 minutes on each side or until golden brown.

Variation: Omit the provolone and roasted vegetables and use mozzarella and fresh tomato slices.

Chicken Almond Wrap

This Mediterranean twist on chicken salad will become a fall favorite. The mixture is held together with a yogurt dressing that has a hint of bright lemon zest.

Yield:	Prep time:	Cook time:	Serving size:
6 servings	20 minutes	20 minutes	½ lavash per serving

Each serving has:			
290 calories	14 g total fat	3 g saturated fat	11 g protein
31 g carbohydrates	3 g fiber	15 mg cholesterol	580 mg sodium

8 oz. boneless, skinless chicken breast

2 tsp. extra-virgin olive oil

½ tsp. kosher salt

¼ tsp. freshly ground black pepper

¼ cup plain Greek yogurt

1 clove garlic, finely minced

1 tsp. spicy brown mustard

1 tsp. honey

1 tsp. lemon zest

½ cup celery, finely diced

1 TB. red onion, finely minced

1 tsp. fresh mint, finely chopped

½ cup red grapes, halved

1 cup Savoy cabbage, finely shredded

¼ cup slivered almonds, toasted

3 lavash-style flatbreads

1½ cups lettuce spring mix

1. Coat chicken breast with 1 teaspoon olive oil. Sprinkle with ¼ teaspoon salt and ⅛ teaspoon pepper. Grill over medium heat for 8 to 10 minutes per side or until internal temperature of 165°F is measured on a meat thermometer in thickest part of breast. Remove from grill and let rest 5 minutes.

2. In a small bowl, combine yogurt, garlic, mustard, honey, lemon zest, and remaining 1 teaspoon olive oil. Mix well.

3. Dice chicken into ½-inch cubes.

4. In a large bowl, combine chicken, celery, onion, mint, grapes, cabbage, remaining ¼ teaspoon salt, remaining ⅛ teaspoon pepper, and almonds. Mix well.

5. Add yogurt mixture to chicken mixture and mix well. Refrigerate 30 minutes to meld flavors.

6. Place 1 cup of chicken mixture on each flatbread. Add ½ cup lettuce greens and roll up. Cut in half and serve.

Mushroom, Artichoke, and Arugula Flatbread

The addition of arugula lends a nice, peppery bite to this fall flatbread dish.

Yield:	Prep time:	Cook time:	Serving size:
1 flatbread	10 minutes	13 to 15 minutes	¼ flatbread

Each serving has:			
140 calories	7 g total fat	1.5 g saturated fat	5 g protein
14 g carbohydrates	2 g fiber	5 mg cholesterol	290 mg sodium

1 TB. extra-virgin olive oil

¼ cup onion, finely diced

1 cup baby portobello mushrooms, sliced

¼ tsp. dried oregano

⅓ cup artichoke quarters in spring water, drained

1 clove garlic, finely minced

6 pitted Kalamata olives, halved

2 TB. white wine

⅛ tsp. freshly ground black pepper

1 (3-oz.) flatbread

½ oz. Parmesan cheese, freshly grated

½ cup fresh arugula leaves

1. Preheat oven to 400°F.

2. In a large sauté pan over medium heat, add oil. When heated, add onions, mushrooms, and oregano. Cook for 5 minutes, stirring occasionally.

3. Add artichokes, garlic, olives, wine, and pepper. Cook for 2 minutes or until wine has evaporated.

4. Place flatbread on an oiled sheet pan. Top with warm mushroom mixture, distributing evenly over bread. Sprinkle ¼ ounce Parmesan cheese on top of the mixture.

5. Bake for 8 to 10 minutes. Remove and top with arugula and remaining ¼ ounce Parmesan cheese. Garnish with additional black pepper and a drizzle of extra-virgin olive oil.

Mouthwatering Entrées

In This Chapter

- Fish and seafood made easy
- Pasta—always a kitchen staple
- Meat the Mediterranean way
- Yummy recipes

Fish receives extra recognition in the Mediterranean diet. In fact, you need to work on getting at least two servings or more each week to get the omega-3 fatty acids you need for good health. Fish and shellfish can be grilled, pan-fried, baked, or put into a stew. Many varieties are available at your local market that are flash-frozen and individually packaged, allowing you to cook only what you need. The recipes in this chapter are easy to make and will help you find tasty ways to include more fish in your weekly menu plans.

Pasta, especially the whole-grain variety, is so versatile and healthy that your kitchen should never be without it. With a basic tomato sauce, pesto, or a little drizzle of a good-quality extra-virgin olive oil combined with shaved Parmesan and freshly ground black pepper, you have the basis of a delicious and nutritious meal. Pasta is typically made from semolina flour (a refined flour) but whole grains such as brown rice pastas, quinoa pastas, and whole-wheat pastas are preferred in the Mediterranean for their higher protein, fiber, vitamin, and mineral content. Try experimenting to find a brand and type you like.

Chicken is the most commonly consumed poultry in Mediterranean cooking and is delicious either hot or cold. If you have had trouble producing a moist chicken breast, you are probably overcooking it. Cook chicken breast to an internal temperature of 165°F—you will produce moist and juicy meat every time.

The yummy recipes in this chapter span all of the seasons and use fresh, seasonal ingredients. Use the recipes in season or whenever you like!

Fish Stew

A light and flavorful stew of tender fish in a savory broth with a hint of spiciness from the red pepper flakes, perfect for a fall dish.

Yield:	Prep time:	Cook time:	Serving size:
8 cups	20 minutes	40 minutes	1 cup

Each serving has:			
210 calories	7 g total fat	1 g saturated fat	22 g protein
9 g carbohydrates	2 g fiber	85 mg cholesterol	440 mg sodium

3 TB. extra-virgin olive oil

4 cloves garlic, thinly sliced

1 large onion, thinly sliced

1 small fennel bulb, bulb only, thinly sliced

1 TB. frozen orange juice concentrate, thawed

1 (14-oz.) can diced tomatoes

½ tsp. red pepper flakes

1 cup dry white wine

5 cups bottled clam juice (or use seafood stock)

2 lb. seafood (use any firm white fish or any shellfish, such as cod, halibut, sole, tilapia, shrimp, clams, or mussels)

1. In a large pot over medium heat, add olive oil.

2. When oil is hot, add garlic, onion, and fennel. Cook for 5 to 10 minutes until beginning to brown.

3. Add orange juice concentrate, tomatoes, red pepper flakes, wine, and clam juice.

4. Bring to a boil then reduce heat to simmer and simmer 30 minutes.

5. While broth is simmering, cut fish into bite-size pieces.

6. Raise heat to medium and add fish (do not add shellfish at this time). Cook for 2 minutes.

7. Add shellfish and cook 5 minutes, or until shells begin to open. Discard any that do not open.

Pan-Seared Orange Scallops

In this summery dish, orange adds a sweet flavor, which intensifies the natural sweetness of the scallops.

Yield:	Prep time:	Cook time:	Serving size:
4 servings	20 minutes	10 minutes	1 cup salad greens, 3 scallops

Each serving has:			
560 calories	43 g total fat	6 g saturated fat	22 g protein
26 g carbohydrates	7 g fiber	35 mg cholesterol	360 mg sodium

3 medium-size oranges

⅛ cup white balsamic vinegar

1 clove garlic, finely minced

1 tsp. Dijon mustard

¼ tsp. kosher salt

½ cup plus 2 TB. extra-virgin olive oil

2 TB. all-purpose flour

1 lb. sea scallops, size U10 (see the Healthy Morsels sidebar)

½ tsp. chopped fresh oregano leaves

4 cups packed mixed salad greens

1 avocado, peeled and diced

1. Zest 1 orange to measure ¼ teaspoon zest and set the orange aside. Juice the remaining 2 oranges to make ½ cup of orange juice.

2. In a small bowl, make salad dressing by combining zest, balsamic vinegar, garlic, Dijon mustard, ⅛ teaspoon salt, and ¼ cup of the orange juice. Discard or save the remaining orange juice for another use. Slowly whisk in ½ cup olive oil. Whisk until combined well, set aside.

3. Cut remaining (zested) orange into segments. On a cutting board, cut off top and bottom of orange. Place orange cut side down on the cutting board. Cut off skin and white pith, slicing around orange from top to bottom. Holding orange over a bowl to catch any juices, cut segments out of orange, leaving the membrane between each section behind. Squeeze the membrane to extract remaining juice. Set orange segments aside.

4. In a large nonstick skillet over medium heat, add remaining 2 tablespoons olive oil.

5. While oil is heating, place flour in a shallow dish. Dredge top and bottom of the scallops in flour, shaking off any excess.

6. When oil is hot, add half of scallops one at a time. Cook for 2 to 3 minutes. Do not move the scallops while they are cooking so they develop a brown crust. Turn scallops over when golden brown and cook another 2 to 3 minutes. Scallops are done when the side of the scallop is all white, with no translucence in the middle.

7. Remove scallops to plate and cover with aluminum foil. If needed, add additional olive oil and cook second batch of scallops in the same manner.

8. Add to hot skillet the remaining ¼ cup orange juice and remaining ⅛ teaspoon salt. Cook 1 to 2 minutes or until reduced by half and liquid resembles a glaze. Remove from heat and stir in oregano.

9. In a large bowl, add salad greens, reserved orange sections, and avocado. Add salad dressing and toss to combine.

10. Divide salad mixture between 4 plates. Top each with 3 scallops. Drizzle each plate with pan sauce.

HEALTHY MORSELS

The scallops called for in this recipe are U10, which refers to the number of scallops in a pound. The *U* means *under,* so U10 means fewer than 10 scallops per pound. The larger the number is, the smaller the scallop.

Sole Florentine

Sole is a mild-flavored white fish that pairs well with the tomatoes of summer and spinach.

Yield:	Prep time:	Cook time:	Serving size:
4 servings	15 minutes	25 to 30 minutes	1 fillet
Each serving has:			
140 calories	5 g total fat	1 g saturated fat	22 g protein
2 g carbohydrates	0 g fiber	55 mg cholesterol	220 mg sodium

½ cup tomatoes, diced

1 clove garlic, minced

1 TB. minced shallot

1 cup chopped fresh spinach

¼ tsp. kosher salt

1 TB. extra-virgin olive oil

4 (4-oz.) sole fillets

Freshly ground black pepper to taste

1 TB. finely chopped fresh parsley

1 lemon, cut into 4 wedges

1. Preheat oven to 350°F.

2. In a small bowl, combine tomatoes, garlic, shallot, spinach, salt, and olive oil.

3. Place one sole fillet on cutting board. Place 1 tablespoon of spinach-tomato mixture on bottom half of fillet. Roll fillet up toward the top so tomato mixture is in the center of fillet. Place seam side down in a greased baking dish. Continue with three remaining fillets. Line fish against each other to prevent unrolling.

4. Pour any additional spinach-tomato mixture over the tops of fillets.

5. Bake at 350°F for 25 to 30 minutes or until fish flakes easily.

6. Garnish with additional salt, pepper, parsley, and lemon wedges.

Almond-Crusted Barramundi

Ground almonds and breadcrumbs lend a pleasing crunch to this spring baked fish entrée. Barramundi is a firm white fish native to northern Australia and southeast Asia. It is very rich in omega-3 fatty acids.

Yield:	Prep time:	Cook time:	Serving size:
4 servings	15 minutes	15 minutes	1 fillet

Each serving has:			
310 calories	14 g total fat	1.5 g saturated fat	27 g protein
20 g carbohydrates	3 g fiber	40 mg cholesterol	270 mg sodium

⅓ cup whole almonds	Zest of one lemon
1 clove garlic	2 TB. Italian breadcrumbs
¼ tsp. freshly ground black pepper	4 (3-oz.) barramundi fillets (or any firm white fish such as snapper, mullet, or halibut)
1 TB. Dijon mustard	
2 TB. honey	
1 TB. extra-virgin olive oil	1 lemon, cut into 4 wedges

1. Preheat oven to 375°F.

2. In the bowl of a food processor, combine almonds, garlic, and pepper. Pulse just until mixture is finely chopped. If you overmix it you will make almond butter.

3. In a small mixing bowl, combine Dijon mustard, honey, olive oil, and lemon zest. Mix well.

4. In another small bowl, combine breadcrumbs with almond mixture.

5. Coat fish in Dijon mustard mixture, then pat almond mixture into fillets, coating each side well.

6. Bake at 375°F for 15 minutes or until fish flakes easily.

7. Serve with a lemon wedge.

Salmon Fennel Bundles

Fennel gives this winter dish a light anise flavor.

Yield:	Prep time:	Cook time:	Serving size:
4 servings	10 minutes	15 minutes	1 fillet

Each serving has:			
390 calories	25 g total fat	3.5 g saturated fat	35 g protein
5 g carbohydrates	2 g fiber	95 mg cholesterol	250 mg sodium

2 TB. freshly squeezed lemon juice	2 TB. dry white wine
¼ cup extra-virgin olive oil	1 fennel bulb
¼ tsp. dried basil	4 (6-oz.) salmon fillets, skin removed
⅛ tsp. salt	
⅛ tsp. freshly ground black pepper	4 tsp. capers

1. Preheat oven to 350°F.

2. In a small bowl, combine lemon juice, olive oil, basil, salt, pepper, and wine. Mix well.

3. Remove green stalks and fronds from fennel bulb. Slice fennel bulb in half through the center of the root. Cut out hard, triangle-shaped core and discard. Slice fennel thinly.

4. Cut 4 pieces of aluminum foil approximately 12 inches long. In the center of each foil piece, place ¼ of sliced fennel.

5. Place 1 salmon fillet on top of each fennel portion.

6. Spoon about 2 tablespoons of lemon mixture over each salmon fillet. Add 1 teaspoon capers on top of each fillet.

7. Seal each packet tightly and bake for 15 minutes. Remove from oven and let rest 5 minutes before opening.

TO YOUR HEALTH

Cooking the salmon inside an aluminum packet with liquid steams the fish, leaving it very moist. You can prepare the packets ahead of time and then when you are ready, pop them in the oven.

Spicy Tomato Sauce with Linguine

Red pepper flakes give this tomato sauce a spicy kick. This summer recipe uses pantry ingredients so it can be made at any time. It also freezes well.

Yield:	Prep time:	Cook time:	Serving size:
About 3½ cups	10 minutes	20 minutes	½ cup

Each serving has:			
200 calories	3 g total fat	0 g saturated fat	6 g protein
36 g carbohydrates	2 g fiber	0 mg cholesterol	190 mg sodium

1 TB. extra-virgin olive oil

½ cup diced onion

½ tsp. kosher salt

2 cloves garlic, finely minced

1 TB. tomato paste

1 tsp. balsamic vinegar

2 (14.5-oz.) cans diced tomatoes, no salt added

1 tsp. Italian seasoning

¼ tsp. crushed red pepper flakes

¼ tsp. freshly ground black pepper

8 oz. uncooked linguine

Freshly shaved Parmesan cheese

1. In a large saucepan over medium heat, add olive oil.

2. When oil is hot, add onion and salt. Cook for 5 minutes, stirring occasionally.

3. Add garlic, tomato paste, and balsamic vinegar. Mix well and sauté for 1 minute.

4. Add tomatoes with liquid, Italian seasoning, red pepper flakes, and black pepper. Simmer for 20 minutes, stirring occasionally.

5. Fill a large pot ⅔ full with water, add salt, and place over medium-high heat. Bring to a boil, add linguine, and cook according to package directions. Drain pasta.

6. Serve ½ cup sauce with ½ cup pasta. Garnish with freshly shaved Parmesan cheese.

Variation: Add your favorite protein such as shrimp or chicken.

Angel Hair Pasta with Pesto, Mushrooms, and Arugula

Peppery arugula adds a nice contrast to the sweet basil pesto in this summer dish.

Yield:	Prep time:	Cook time:	Serving size:
6 cups	15 minutes	10 minutes	1 cup

Each serving has:			
260 calories	11 g total fat	2 g saturated fat	8 g protein
32 g carbohydrates	2 g fiber	5 mg cholesterol	60 mg sodium

1 tsp. kosher salt	8 oz. baby portobello mushrooms, sliced
8 oz. uncooked angel hair pasta (may also be labeled as capellini)	⅓ cup Pesto (recipe in Chapter 17)
1 TB. extra-virgin olive oil	3 cups arugula
½ cup diced onion	Freshly shaved Parmesan cheese

1. Fill a large pot ⅔ full with water, add salt, and place over medium-high heat. Bring to a boil, add pasta, and cook according to package directions. Drain pasta.

2. In a large skillet over medium heat, add olive oil.

3. When oil is hot, add onion and cook for 4 minutes until onion is soft.

4. Add mushrooms and cook for 5 minutes or until liquid released from mushrooms has evaporated. Remove pan from heat.

5. In a large bowl, toss pasta with Pesto.

6. Add arugula to the skillet containing mushroom mixture and toss well. Arugula should be slightly wilted.

7. Place pesto angel hair pasta mixture on a large serving platter or on individual plates and top with arugula mushroom mixture.

8. Garnish with shaved Parmesan cheese.

Variation: Use the same amount of baby spinach leaves instead of arugula.

Lamb Patties and Pasta

Lamb patties are a great alternative to the usual beef patties we are all familiar with. Surprise your guests this spring with these savory patties.

Yield:	Prep time:	Cook time:	Serving size:
4 servings	20 minutes	15 minutes	3 patties per portion, 1 cup pasta

Each serving has:			
660 calories	38 g total fat	15 g saturated fat	860 mg sodium
42 g carbohydrates	4 g fiber	135 mg cholesterol	38 g protein

1 lb. ground lamb

¾ cup finely chopped yellow onion

1 TB. finely minced garlic

¾ tsp. kosher salt

½ tsp. freshly ground black pepper

8 oz. uncooked linguine

1 TB. pine nuts

8 oz. white button mushrooms

¼ cup sun-dried tomatoes, sliced into strips

1 cup fresh baby spinach

1 cup arugula

4 oz. manchego cheese, shredded (about 1 cup)

1. In a medium bowl, combine ground lamb, ½ cup onion, garlic, ½ teaspoon salt, and ¼ teaspoon pepper. Mix well.

2. Form mixture into 12 patties that are about 2 inches in diameter and ¾-inch thick.

3. Heat a large nonstick skillet over medium heat. Add patties and cook 3 to 4 minutes on each side until lightly browned and cooked through. Transfer patties to a plate and cover with foil to keep warm. Retain the pan and its juices.

4. Fill a large pot ⅔ full with water, add salt, and place over medium-high heat. Bring to a boil, add linguine, and cook according to package directions. Drain linguine.

5. Toast pine nuts over medium heat in a small skillet for 3 to 4 minutes while the pasta is cooking. Nuts should be lightly browned. Remove nuts from pan and set aside.

6. Wash mushrooms and discard the stems. Slice into ⅛-inch thick slices.

7. Place the fry pan used to cook the patties with all its juices back over medium heat. When pan is warm, add remaining ¼ cup onion, sliced mushrooms, sun-dried tomatoes, remaining ¼ teaspoon salt, and remaining ¼ teaspoon pepper. Cook for 4 minutes, stirring occasionally.

8. Add spinach and arugula to mushroom mixture. Remove from the heat and mix well. Greens should be slightly wilted. Add pine nuts and pasta. Mix well.

9. Place 1 cup pasta mixture and 3 lamb patties on each plate. Garnish with manchego cheese. Serve immediately.

Variation: Manchego cheese is a Spanish sheep's milk cheese. If you can't find it, you can substitute pecorino or Parmesan. Also feel free to use only spinach instead of spinach and arugula.

TO YOUR HEALTH

Make extra lamb patties and freeze for another time. These patties are also great stuffed in a pita.

Lamb Shanks

This is a classic hearty spring dish with a rich meaty sauce.

Yield:	Prep time:	Cook time:	Serving size:
4 servings	20 minutes	2¼ hours	1 shank with ½ cup sauce

Each serving has:			
550 calories	37 g total fat	10 g saturated fat	26 g protein
26 g carbohydrates	4 g fiber	80 mg cholesterol	170 mg sodium

4 (4-oz.) lamb shanks	⅓ cup tomato paste
¼ cup all-purpose flour	6 cloves garlic, finely minced
¼ cup plus 2 TB. extra-virgin olive oil	½ tsp. dried oregano
2 stalks celery, sliced ¼-inch thick	½ tsp. dried rosemary
1½ cups carrots (about 2 to 3 large), sliced ¼-inch thick	¼ tsp. freshly ground black pepper
2 cups chopped onion	2 cups dry red wine
	4 cups beef broth
	2 bay leaves

1. Dredge lamb shanks with flour and shake off excess.

2. In large 8-quart pot, add ¼ cup oil. When oil is hot, brown shanks, cooking 3 to 4 minutes per side. Depending on size of shanks, you may only be able to brown two at one time.

3. When all shanks are browned, discard oil and clean pot. Next, add remaining 2 tablespoons olive oil to cleaned pot and heat over medium heat. Add celery, carrots, and onion. Cook 10 minutes.

4. Add tomato paste, garlic, oregano, rosemary, and pepper. Cook for 3 minutes, stirring occasionally.

5. Add wine, broth, and bay leaves. Stir well. Add lamb shanks and bring to a boil.

6. Remove from heat and cover pot. Bake in 325°F oven for 2 hours or until tender.

7. Skim oil from surface.

8. Serve one shank and ½ cup sauce per person along with couscous, rice, polenta, or mashed potatoes, if desired.

Crispy Turkey Cutlets

These cutlets have a nice crunch from the breadcrumb coating, which is laced with Parmesan cheese. It's the perfect comfort food during the cold winter months.

Yield:	Prep time:	Cook time:	Serving size:
4 servings	20 minutes	15 minutes	4 ounces

Each serving has:			
320 calories	14 g total fat	4 g saturated fat	37 g protein
12 g carbohydrates	1 g fiber	160 mg cholesterol	580 mg sodium

1 lb. boneless, skinless turkey breast

½ cup freshly grated Parmesan cheese

½ cup Italian-seasoned bread-crumbs

⅛ tsp. kosher salt

⅛ tsp. freshly ground black pepper

2 eggs, beaten

2 TB. extra-virgin olive oil

1 TB. finely chopped fresh parsley

1 lemon, cut into 4 wedges

1. Slice turkey breast into 4 equally sized pieces.

2. Place one piece on a cutting board and cover with plastic wrap. Using a meat mallet, pound until turkey is ¼-inch thick. Set aside and repeat until all pieces are pounded out.

3. In a small bowl, combine Parmesan cheese, breadcrumbs, salt, and pepper. Pour onto a large plate.

4. Dip each turkey piece into beaten eggs, and then coat with breadcrumbs on each side. Repeat with the remaining turkey.

5. In large skillet over medium heat, add oil. When hot, add two breaded turkey breasts and cook for 2 minutes on each side or until golden brown. Reduce heat and continue cooking if they brown too quickly or the turkey is still pink inside. Cook breast to an internal temperature of 165°F. Repeat for other two breasts.

6. Garnish each serving with parsley and a lemon wedge.

TO YOUR HEALTH

If you have any leftover bread that has gone stale, make your own bread-crumbs. Dry the bread out completely by leaving it uncovered on a sheet pan and then toss in a food processor and process until fine. For this recipe, add ¼ teaspoon each of garlic powder, oregano, basil, and salt.

Chicken Piccata

This great chicken dish has a refreshing hint of lemon and piquant capers, perfect for spring.

Yield:	Prep time:	Cook time:	Serving size:
4 servings	20 minutes	20 minutes	4 ounces chicken breast, ¼ cup sauce, ¼ cup spinach leaves

Each serving has:			
390 calories	22 g total fat	4.5 g saturated fat	19 g protein
29 g carbohydrates	3 g fiber	45 mg cholesterol	890 mg sodium

4 (4-oz.) boneless, skinless chicken breasts

¼ cup all-purpose flour

¼ tsp. kosher salt

¼ tsp. freshly ground black pepper

1 TB. extra-virgin olive oil

1 cup white onion (about 1 onion), finely diced

2 TB. white wine or chicken broth

1 TB. freshly squeezed lemon juice

½ cup low-sodium chicken broth

1 clove garlic, finely minced

3 TB. capers

1 cup baby spinach leaves

1 freezer-safe bag or plastic wrap

1 TB. finely chopped fresh parsley

1. Place chicken breasts into a freezer-safe bag or cover with 2 layers of plastic wrap and place on a cutting board. Pound each chicken breast with a meat pounder or a heavy skillet until ½-inch thick.

2. On a large, shallow plate, combine flour, salt, and pepper. Mix well. Dredge each chicken breast in flour coating. Shake off any extra flour. In a large skillet over medium heat, add olive oil. When oil is hot, add chicken breasts and cook for 4 to 6 minutes per side or until slightly golden in color. Reduce heat and continue cooking if they brown too quickly or the chicken is still pink inside. Cook breast to an internal temperature of 165°F.

3. Transfer chicken to a plate and cover with aluminum foil to keep warm.

4. Add onion to the skillet and cook for 1 minute. Add wine, lemon juice, broth, garlic, and capers. Cook for 5 to 7 minutes until liquid has reduced by half and mixture has thickened slightly. Place spinach leaves on a platter and top with chicken. Divide pan sauce equally, pouring over chicken. Garnish with parsley.

Tasty Side Dishes

In This Chapter

- Vegetables—underrated and overcooked
- Legumes, canned or cooked?
- Grains to round out your meals
- Scrumptious recipes

Combining vegetables, legumes, and grains can make a powerfully nutritious side dish—and even a complete meal. The different flavors and textures make the possible combinations endless. There is a vegetable for every season. Make it a point each month to try a new vegetable recipe, such as those in this chapter, and see if it moves to the top of your shopping list. Something your family has never tried may just become their new favorite!

Canned and dried beans are a must for every kitchen pantry. Serve them cold in a salad or puréed into a creamy dip, or add them to soups, casseroles, stews, or even your favorite steamed veggie. Some versatile beans to keep on hand are garbanzo beans, red kidney beans, and cannellini beans, although any type of bean you enjoy should be in your cupboard. On days when you have more time in your schedule, soak a pot of dried beans before you go to bed. The next day, drain the water and cook the beans. It's a great way to use up any leftover vegetables or meat, which you can add to your pot of beans during the last hour of cooking.

Whole grains are easy to find at your local market. They combine well with many different foods and make a great base for vegetables, herbs, and spices. Cook up a batch of bulgur, polenta, quinoa, or barley. Add a little onion, garlic, or any vegetable you have on hand for a simple and healthy dish.

The scrumptious recipes in this chapter span all of the seasons and use fresh, seasonal ingredients. Use the recipes in season or whenever you like!

Zucchini and Walnuts

Zucchini takes on a new life with walnuts and sweet mint in this fragrant, delicious mixture, perfect on a summer day.

Yield:	Prep time:	Cook time:	Serving size:
3 cups	15 minutes	7 minutes	½ cup

Each serving has:			
70 calories	5 g total fat	0.5 g saturated fat	1 g protein
4 g carbohydrates	1 g fiber	0 mg cholesterol	85 mg sodium

2 large zucchini (about 2¼ cups sliced)

1 TB. extra-virgin olive oil

½ cup finely diced onion

1 cup sliced baby portobello mushrooms

¼ tsp. kosher salt

⅛ tsp. freshly ground black pepper

3 TB. finely chopped walnuts

2 tsp. finely chopped mint leaves

1. Slice zucchini in half lengthwise. Cut each half lengthwise again so you have 4 pieces. Slice across into ¼-inch slices.

2. In a large skillet over medium heat, add oil. When oil is hot, add onion. Cook, stirring occasionally, for 1 minute.

3. Add mushrooms, zucchini, salt, and pepper. Cook for 3 minutes, stirring occasionally. Add walnuts and mint and cook for 1 minute. Remove from heat and serve.

Variation: Use any type of mushroom you have available. Also try using other nuts such as pecans, cashews, or almonds.

Two-Cheese Risotto

Classic risotto is rich, creamy, and has a souplike consistency. It's the perfect comfort food on a cold winter day.

Yield:	Prep time:	Cook time:	Serving size:
8 cups	10 minutes	40 minutes	½ cup
Each serving has:			
175 calories	5 g total fat	1.5 g saturated fat	7 g protein
25 g carbohydrates	1 g fiber	10 mg cholesterol	180 mg sodium

3 TB. extra-virgin olive oil

1 cup onion (about 1), finely chopped

2 cloves garlic, finely chopped

8 cups low-sodium chicken broth

16 oz. arborio rice

½ cup white wine

1 cup freshly grated Parmesan cheese

¼ cup freshly grated asiago cheese

½ tsp. kosher salt

1. In a small skillet over medium heat, add 1 tablespoon olive oil. When hot, add onions and sauté 8 minutes. Add garlic and cook 2 minutes more. Remove from heat.

2. In a large pot over low heat, add broth and bring to a simmer.

3. In a 6-quart pot over medium heat, add remaining 2 tablespoons olive oil. When oil is hot, add rice. Cook 7 minutes, stirring constantly to prevent sticking.

4. Add wine to hot rice and continue stirring until all wine has evaporated.

5. Add 1 ladle full of warm broth (about ½ cup) to rice and constantly stir with a wooden spoon or heat safe spatula until the rice has absorbed all of the liquid. Repeat, adding 1 ladle of broth each time, stirring constantly. Continue until rice will not absorb any more liquid. This will take 20 to 25 minutes.

6. Add sautéed onion mixture to rice.

7. Rice should have a thick, souplike consistency. Remove from heat and add Parmesan cheese, asiago cheese, and salt. Stir to combine.

Variation: Sauté 8 ounces sliced mushrooms along with the onions.

GOOD TO KNOW

It is important to use the right kind of rice when making risotto. Arborio is the traditional rice for risotto and is a high-starch, short-grained rice. If you were to use a regular long-grain rice, the recipe would lose its creamy consistency.

Sautéed Spinach and Mushrooms

Garlic permeates the spinach and mushrooms to create a perfect base for fish or chicken. It also makes for a delicious summer side dish.

Yield:	Prep time:	Cook time:	Serving size:
2 cups	10 minutes	6 minutes	½ cup

Each serving has:			
100 calories	6 g total fat	2 g saturated fat	6 g protein
10 g carbohydrates	4 g fiber	5 mg cholesterol	270 mg sodium

1 TB. extra-virgin olive oil	¼ tsp. freshly ground black pepper
4 cloves garlic, finely minced	10 cups spinach leaves
8 oz. mushrooms, sliced	1 oz. freshly grated Parmesan cheese
⅛ tsp. kosher salt	

1. In a large skillet over medium heat, add olive oil.

2. When oil is hot, add garlic, mushrooms, salt, and pepper. Cook for 5 minutes.

3. Add spinach to skillet and stir continuously for 1 minute or until spinach is wilted.

4. Remove from heat and stir in Parmesan cheese.

Rosemary Garlic Potatoes

Flavored with the piney, floral taste of rosemary, these potatoes smell and taste delicious and make the perfect winter side dish!

Yield:	Prep time:	Cook time:	Serving size:
2 cups	10 minutes	30 minutes	½ cup

Each serving has:			
140 calories	7 g total fat	1 g saturated fat	2 g protein
19 g carbohydrates	2 g fiber	0 mg cholesterol	125 mg sodium

1 lb. red potatoes, unpeeled and scrubbed well

2 TB. extra-virgin olive oil

1 tsp. finely minced fresh rosemary leaves

2 cloves garlic, finely minced

¼ tsp. kosher salt

⅛ tsp. freshly ground black pepper

1. Preheat oven to 400°F.

2. Cut potatoes into quarters.

3. In a large bowl, combine olive oil, rosemary, garlic, salt, and pepper.

4. Toss potatoes in oil mixture. Transfer to a sheet pan.

5. Bake for 30 minutes or until golden brown, stirring occasionally.

Curried Cauliflower

This dish is a sweet and savory winter dish with crunchy almonds and golden, sweet raisins.

Yield:	Prep time:	Cook time:	Serving size:
3 cups	15 minutes	30 minutes	½ cup

Each serving has:			
120 calories	7 g total fat	1 g saturated fat	3 g protein
14 g carbohydrates	3 g fiber	0 mg cholesterol	190 mg sodium

1 medium head cauliflower

2 TB. extra-virgin olive oil

½ tsp. kosher salt

⅛ tsp. freshly ground black pepper

2 cloves garlic, finely minced

1 tsp. curry powder

1 medium red onion, thinly sliced

¼ cup golden raisins

¼ cup slivered almonds, toasted

1. Preheat oven to 350°F.

2. Core cauliflower by cutting out the triangular shape at the base of the head after slicing the head in half. Separate into florets. Cut large pieces, if necessary, so all pieces are approximately the same size.

3. In a large bowl, combine oil, salt, pepper, garlic, and curry powder. Mix well.

4. Add cauliflower, onion, and raisins to oil mixture and mix thoroughly.

5. Transfer cauliflower mixture to a 9×9 casserole dish. Add 2 tablespoons water.

6. Bake for 30 minutes or until cauliflower is tender, stirring occasionally. Remove from oven and sprinkle with almonds.

Lemon Kale Ribbons

Red pepper flakes and garlic give a nice kick to leafy green kale, perfect for summer.

Yield:	Prep time:	Cook time:	Serving size:
2 cups	15 minutes	3 minutes	½ cup

Each serving has:			
100 calories	7 g total fat	1 g saturated fat	2 g protein
7 g carbohydrates	1 g fiber	0 mg cholesterol	150 mg sodium

8 oz. fresh kale, rinsed	⅛ tsp. crushed red pepper flakes
2 TB. extra-virgin olive oil	1 TB. freshly squeezed lemon juice
1 TB. finely minced shallot	¼ tsp. kosher salt
4 cloves garlic, finely sliced	⅛ tsp. freshly ground black pepper

1. Cut away the tough center stalks of the kale leaves. Slice leaves into ¼-inch strips.

2. In a large skillet over medium heat, add oil.

3. When oil is hot, add shallot, garlic, and red pepper flakes and cook 1 minute.

4. Add kale and cook 2 minutes, stirring constantly.

5. Remove from heat and add lemon juice, salt, and pepper. Mix well to combine.

Variation: Cook a slice of pancetta or bacon and then cook the shallots and garlic in the reserved oil to add flavor. Use the crispy pancetta or bacon crumbled as a garnish.

Minted Peas with Pancetta

Peas get a spring pick-me-up with the addition of refreshing fresh mint and pancetta.

Yield:	Prep time:	Cook time:	Serving size:
1½ cups	5 minutes	6 minutes	½ cup

Each serving has:			
140 calories	7 g total fat	2 g saturated fat	7 g protein
14 g carbohydrates	4 g fiber	10 mg cholesterol	300 mg sodium

1½ oz. pancetta (unsmoked bacon), diced

2 TB. finely diced shallots

10 oz. frozen peas, thawed

1 TB. finely sliced, fresh mint leaves

⅛ tsp. kosher salt

⅛ tsp. freshly ground black pepper

1. In a large skillet over medium heat, cook pancetta for 3 minutes or until lightly browned.

2. Add shallots to the pan and cook for 1 minute.

3. Add peas and cook 2 minutes or until warmed through, stirring occasionally.

4. Remove from heat and add mint, salt, and pepper.

Variation: Substitute bacon if you can't find the pancetta.

Pickled Asparagus

This crisp and tangy asparagus is delicious eaten alone or added to a spring salad.

Yield:	Prep time:	Cook time:	Serving size:
8 servings	10 minutes	15 minutes	⅛ recipe

Each serving has:			
40 calories	0 g total fat	0 g saturated fat	1 g protein
7 g carbohydrates	1 g fiber	0 mg cholesterol	720 mg sodium

1 lb. fresh asparagus	1 heaping tsp. pickling spices
1½ cups distilled white vinegar	1 tsp. crushed red pepper flakes
3 TB. sugar	1 sprig fresh dill
3 tsp. kosher salt	1 garlic clove, sliced

1. Wash asparagus and trim the tough ends.

2. Fill a large pot ¾ full of water and bring to a boil over high heat. Add asparagus and blanch for 1 minute. Immediately transfer asparagus to a large bowl of ice water to cool, allowing it to keep its bright green color.

3. In a small pot over medium heat, add 1½ cups water, vinegar, sugar, salt, pickling spices, red pepper flakes, and dill. Cook for 4 minutes, stirring occasionally until sugar is dissolved. Cool completely.

4. Pack asparagus and garlic slices into a canning jar or any glass container that can be covered tightly. Pour vinegar mixture into jar. Chill overnight in the refrigerator and keep refrigerated. Consume within one week.

Variation: Add a few small whole or sliced peppers such as banana peppers along with the asparagus.

Bean and Vegetable Patties

The cornmeal in this fall recipe adds a pleasing sweetness and a crispy texture. This recipe can be used as an entrée or appetizer. For an appetizer, make smaller patties and serve with a garlic aioli (a strongly flavored garlic mayonnaise).

Yield:	Prep time:	Cook time:	Serving size:
15 patties	15 minutes	30 minutes	1 patty

Each serving has:			
140 calories	5 g total fat	1 g saturated fat	5 g protein
19 g carbohydrates	3 g fiber	30 mg cholesterol	240 mg sodium

1 (15-oz.) can red kidney beans, rinsed and drained	¼ tsp. freshly ground black pepper
1 large red bell pepper, cored and chopped	4 TB. extra-virgin olive oil, plus more for garnish
2 stalks celery, roughly chopped	¾ cup cornmeal
1 small zucchini, roughly chopped	1 cup all-purpose flour
¼ cup fresh parsley leaves	¼ cup freshly grated Parmesan cheese plus more for garnish
1 clove garlic	2 eggs, beaten
½ red onion, roughly chopped	Diced fresh tomatoes for garnish
1 tsp. kosher salt	

1. Preheat oven to 350°F.

2. Place kidney beans into a food processor and pulse until processed but still chunky.

3. Add bell pepper, celery, zucchini, parsley, garlic, onion, salt, pepper, and 3 tablespoons olive oil. Pulse several times until all ingredients are blended. Vegetables should be chunky and uniform in size, but not puréed. Scrape the sides of the processor and pulse until all ingredients are incorporated.

4. In a large mixing bowl, combine cornmeal, flour, and Parmesan cheese.

5. Add bean mixture and egg to cornmeal mixture. Mix well to combine.

6. Measure bean mixture into ¼-cup portions. You may want to coat the measuring cup lightly in oil to help the mixture release. Form each portion into a patty ½-inch thick.

7. In a large skillet over medium heat, add additional 1 tablespoon olive oil. When oil is hot, add 5 to 6 patties to the pan. Do not overcrowd. Cook patties 3 minutes per side or until golden brown. Continue with remaining mixture. You may need to add another tablespoon of olive oil between batches.

8. As patties are cooked, place them on an ungreased cookie sheet. When all patties have been cooked in the skillet, place the cookie sheet in the oven and bake for 15 minutes. Patties will become lighter and rise.

9. Serve with fresh diced tomatoes, a drizzle of olive oil, and freshly grated Parmesan cheese.

Variation: Experiment with the beans in this recipe. Try using garbanzo beans or black-eyed peas.

Panzanella

This easy springtime salad pops with savory goodness from balsamic vinegar, roasted red peppers, and artichoke hearts.

Yield:	Prep time:	Cook time:	Serving size:
9 cups	30 minutes	15–20 minutes	1 cup

Each serving has:			
300 calories	17 g total fat	2 g saturated fat	7 g protein
35 g carbohydrates	3 g fiber	0 mg cholesterol	650 mg sodium

1 French baguette

1 (13.75-oz.) can artichoke hearts packed in water, drained

1 cup diced celery (about 1 large stalk)

½ cup roasted red peppers

¼ cup finely diced red onion

⅓ cup chopped sun-dried tomatoes packed in oil

¼ cup chopped fresh parsley

⅔ cup balsamic vinaigrette

Nonstick spray oil or mister with olive oil

1. Preheat oven to 350°F.

2. Slice baguette into 1-inch cubes. Transfer to a sheet pan and lightly spray the bread with a nonstick cooking oil or a mister with olive oil.

3. Bake for 10 to 15 minutes. Remove from oven and cool. This will help prevent the bread from getting soggy when combined with remaining ingredients.

4. Cut artichoke hearts into bite-size pieces.

5. In a large bowl, combine celery, peppers, onion, tomatoes, parsley, artichoke hearts, and bread cubes, mixing well.

6. Pour balsamic vinaigrette into bowl with bread mixture and toss well to combine. Let rest at room temperature for 30 minutes to distribute flavor or refrigerate overnight.

Variation: Substitute 1 large fresh tomato, chopped; half a cucumber, peeled, seeded, and diced; and ¼ cup chopped basil for the vegetables.

HEALTHY MORSELS

Panzanella or bread salad is popular in the Tuscany region of Italy. They often use stale or leftover bread.

Golden Chard

Chard has a mild flavor that is enhanced in this summer recipe with sweet raisins and a touch of honey.

Yield:	Prep time:	Cook time:	Serving size:
2 cups	10 minutes	6 minutes	½ cup

Each serving has:			
130 calories	6 g total fat	1.5 g saturated fat	2 g protein
18 g carbohydrates	2 g fiber	5 mg cholesterol	410 mg sodium

1 lb. chard (about 1 bunch)	½ tsp. kosher salt
1 slice pancetta (unsmoked bacon), diced	¼ tsp. freshly ground black pepper
1 TB. extra-virgin olive oil	⅓ cup golden raisins
2 TB. finely diced shallots	1 TB. honey

1. Remove the large part of stem from chard leaves and set aside. Slice chard leaves crosswise into ¼-inch ribbons. Chop stems crosswise into ¼-inch pieces and keep separate from leaves.

2. In a large nonstick skillet over medium heat, cook pancetta until crisp.

3. Add olive oil, shallots, chard stems, salt, and pepper. Cook for 5 minutes, stirring occasionally.

4. Add chard leaves, raisins, and honey. Cook for 1 to 3 minutes until chard is soft, stirring frequently. Remove from heat immediately.

Variation: Use bacon in a 1:1 replacement instead of pancetta to add a smoky flavor.

TO YOUR HEALTH

The most common chard in the grocery store is usually Swiss chard with white stems, which is a great choice. At farmers' markets there may be different varieties with beautiful yellow, orange, or red stems. Use any variety you find for this recipe. Remember, the more color, the more phytonutrients!

Sweet Polenta with Sun-Dried Tomatoes

Polenta is ground cornmeal. This recipe adds canned corn, which gives extra sweetness to the polenta. This makes a nice winter dish.

Yield:	Prep time:	Cook time:	Serving size:
12 pieces	5 minutes	25 minutes	1 piece
Each serving has:			
90 calories	3 g total fat	0 g saturated fat	2 g protein
14 g carbohydrates	2 g fiber	0 mg cholesterol	200 mg sodium

1 tsp. kosher salt

1 cup cornmeal

1 (15-oz.) can corn, no added salt, drained

⅓ cup sun-dried tomatoes packed in oil, chopped

2 TB. extra-virgin olive oil

1. In a medium pot over high heat, add 4 cups water and salt. Bring to a boil.

2. When water is boiling, add cornmeal very slowly, whisking constantly. Adding cornmeal too quickly will cause lumps.

3. Once all cornmeal is added, reduce heat to low. You may need to pull the pan off the heat temporarily to prevent splattering until the mixture cools down. Continue to whisk mixture to prevent lumps.

4. Continue whisking mixture over low heat. As cornmeal cooks, it will begin to solidify. It should pull away from the pan cleanly around the 20-minute mark.

5. Add corn and tomatoes. Replace the whisk with a spatula and continue cooking for 5 minutes.

6. You can serve the polenta at this point spooned out like mashed potatoes or chill it and then sauté at a later time.

7. If you plan to chill and sauté at a later time, grease a 9×12 pan with 1 tablespoon olive oil. Evenly spread warm polenta into pan. Refrigerate 3 to 4 hours or overnight.

8. Cut polenta into 12 equal portions and transfer each piece to a sheet pan.

9. Lightly dust the top and bottom of each piece with flour.

10. In a large nonstick skillet over medium heat, add 1 tablespoon olive oil. When oil is hot, add 6 to 8 polenta squares depending on the size of pan. Do not over-crowd. Cook 4 minutes per side or until golden. You may need to add additional olive oil between batches.

11. Remove from pan and serve. Use polenta as a side for any protein foods like chicken, seafood, or lamb.

Variation: If you plan to serve immediately after cooking the polenta, the addition of cheese is a nice accompaniment. Add ½ cup freshly grated Parmesan or Romano cheese and stir to combine.

HEALTHY MORSELS

Freshly cooked polenta is creamy like mashed potatoes or a thick hot cereal, while the formed and sliced version that is sautéed is thick and firm.

Quinoa Pilaf

Quinoa looks a bit like rice but has a fluffy texture and a nice crunch when you bite into it. This dish is good served either hot or cold for a fall-time delight.

Yield:	Prep time:	Cook time:	Serving size:
2 cups	10 minutes	25–30 minutes	½ cup

Each serving has:			
150 calories	7 g total fat	2 g saturated fat	5 g protein
18 g carbohydrates	2 g fiber	10 mg cholesterol	510 mg sodium

½ cup quinoa

1 TB. extra-virgin olive oil

1 garlic clove, minced

⅓ cup chopped yellow bell pepper (about ⅓ of a pepper)

¼ cup chopped scallions, green and white parts

1 cup diced canned tomatoes, with juice

½ tsp. kosher salt

⅛ tsp. freshly ground pepper

4 TB. crumbled feta cheese

4 TB. chopped fresh parsley

1. In a small saucepan, bring 1 cup water to a boil. Add quinoa and return to a boil, then lower the temperature to low and cover.

2. Cook quinoa for 15 to 20 minutes or until water is absorbed.

3. In a medium skillet over medium heat, add the olive oil. When oil is hot, add the garlic and bell pepper and sauté for 2 minutes. Add the scallions and cook for 1 minute.

4. Add tomatoes, cooked quinoa, salt, and pepper. Stir to combine.

5. Cook for 2 minutes or until heated through.

6. Top each serving with 1 tablespoon of feta cheese and parsley.

Variation: Try any combination of vegetables, such as zucchini and cucumbers—or even dried fruit.

Barley and Vegetable Sauté

Barley is a plump, moist grain that takes on the sweet flavors of vegetables, as you'll find in this fall recipe.

Yield:	Prep time:	Cook time:	Serving size:
4 cups	20 minutes	18 minutes	½ cup
Each serving has:			
130 calories	6 g total fat	1 g saturated fat	2 g protein
19 g carbohydrates	3 g fiber	0 mg cholesterol	200 mg sodium

2 TB. extra-virgin olive oil

1 cup diced onion

1 cup sweet potato, peeled, cut into ¼-inch cubes (about 1 medium potato)

2 cups pearl barley, cooked according to package directions

1 cup zucchini, quartered and sliced ⅛-inch thick

1 stalk celery, sliced ⅛-inch thick

2 cloves garlic, minced

1 cup grape tomatoes, halved

¼ tsp. minced fresh sage

½ tsp. minced fresh rosemary leaves

¾ tsp. kosher salt

½ tsp. freshly ground black pepper

¼ cup chopped toasted walnuts

2 TB. chopped fresh parsley

1. In a large nonstick skillet over medium heat, add the olive oil.

2. When oil is hot, add onion and sweet potato cubes. Cook for 10 minutes or until the sweet potatoes are tender.

3. Add cooked barley and stir to combine. Cook for 1 to 2 minutes until the barley is warmed through.

4. Add zucchini, celery, garlic, tomatoes, sage, rosemary, salt, and pepper. Cook for 5 minutes.

5. Garnish with walnuts and parsley, and serve.

Variation: Use any variety of vegetables such as carrots, bell peppers, corn, or leeks.

Delectable Desserts

In This Chapter

- Fruit for every day and in every way
- Versatile nuts for flavor
- The perfect snack combination
- Tempting recipes

You may be used to thinking of fruit as a snack because it's easily portable, but in the Mediterranean fruit is the dessert of choice. It can be as simple as sliced or dried fruit paired with cheese at the end of a meal, or it could be something that takes a little more time to whip up. Add a little fruit to a recipe to add another layer of flavor or remake a dish into something completely new. Look at using fruit in new ways by incorporating it into all of your recipes.

Nuts naturally pair well with fruit. They, too, are a great portable snack. Nuts are best toasted to bring out all their nutty goodness. A variety of recipes and uses have been provided in this chapter to help you learn how to include nuts in a variety of ways every day.

The tempting recipes in this chapter span all of the seasons and use fresh, seasonal ingredients. Use the recipes in season or whenever you like!

Cinnamon Apple Nut Phyllo Rolls

This filling is similar to apple pie, but the rolls have a crunchy pastry crust of phyllo dough. Fall is the perfect time to find apples at their best.

Yield:	Prep time:	Cook time:	Serving size:
6 rolls	30 minutes	15–20 minutes	1 roll

Each serving has:			
270 calories	14 g total fat	2 g saturated fat	2 g protein
38 g carbohydrates	3 g fiber	0 mg cholesterol	95 mg sodium

Juice of one lemon

2 red apples, peeled and cored; cut into ⅛-inch dice

½ cup dark brown sugar

¼ cup walnuts

1 tsp. ground cinnamon

6 sheets frozen phyllo dough, thawed according to package directions

4 TB. olive oil

Confectioners' sugar for garnish

1. Preheat oven to 350°F.

2. In a small bowl, combine lemon juice and diced apples. Toss well to coat the apples.

3. Add brown sugar, walnuts, and cinnamon to the apples. Mix well.

4. Lay out one sheet of phyllo dough lengthwise. Brush with olive oil.

5. Place ¼ cup apple-nut mixture 2 inches from the short end of the phyllo dough sheet. Spread along the short end so that apple mixture is about 1½ inches wide by 5 inches long with the mixture centered between the top and bottom edges of the phyllo dough. Fold the long edges of the phyllo dough sheet toward the middle. Brush with more oil and roll the dough starting at the end with the apple mixture to create a log shape. Repeat for remaining phyllo dough sheets. Brush tops with oil.

6. Bake on a greased cookie sheet for 15 to 20 minutes or until pastry is golden brown.

7. Garnish with confectioners' sugar.

Variation: Use any type of fruit instead of apples, or try almonds or pecans instead of walnuts.

Vanilla Panna Cotta

Real vanilla bean flavors the cream and milk in this simple spring dessert.

Yield:	Prep time:	Cook time:	Serving size:
4 servings	15 minutes	10 minutes	4 ounces

Each serving has:			
160 calories	8 g total fat	5 g saturated fat	5 g protein
18 g carbohydrates	0 g fiber	30 mg cholesterol	50 mg sodium

1¾ cups reduced-fat milk, chilled   ¼ cup heavy whipping cream

2½ tsp. unflavored gelatin granules   ½ vanilla bean

¼ cup sugar   1 cup fresh berries

1. Pour ¼ cup milk into a small bowl. Sprinkle gelatin over milk, stir, and let rest 10 minutes.

2. In a medium pan over low heat, add the remaining 1½ cups milk, sugar, and cream.

3. Cut the vanilla bean lengthwise and scrape seeds out of pod with the blade of a small paring knife. Add seeds and pod to milk mixture.

4. Heat on low for 10 minutes. Do not allow to boil.

5. Add gelatin mixture to warm liquid. Whisk to combine. Cook for 1 to 2 minutes and remove from heat. Discard vanilla bean pod.

6. Pour mixture evenly into 4 1-cup ramekins that have been sprayed with non-stick spray.

7. Refrigerate 2 hours or overnight. To serve, run a knife around inside the ramekin to loosen the panna cotta. Dip the bottom of the ramekin in a bowl of hot water for a few seconds to help release the panna cotta from the dish. Turn ramekin upside down on a plate to release panna cotta.

8. Serve with a side of fresh berries.

Variation: Add citrus zest or other spices like cinnamon. You can omit the heavy cream and just use all milk, but the little bit of cream enhances the texture.

Poached Summer Fruit

Wine and spices add an extra zesty flavor to the sweet summer fruit.

Yield:	Prep time:	Cook time:	Serving size:
4 portions	30 minutes	5 minutes	¼ recipe

Each serving has:			
190 calories	0 g total fat	0 g saturated fat	1 g protein
45 g carbohydrates	5 g fiber	0 mg cholesterol	0 mg sodium

1 bottle (750 ml) white wine

1 cup sugar

1 cinnamon stick

1 lemon, juiced and zested

1 slice fresh ginger root, ½-inch thick

2 pears, peeled, cored, and halved

2 peaches, peeled, pitted, and halved

2 plums, peeled, pitted, and halved

1. In a medium saucepan over medium heat, combine wine, sugar, cinnamon stick, lemon juice and zest, and ginger. Bring to a boil and cook for about 5 minutes or until sugar is dissolved. Reduce heat to a simmer.

2. Add fruit to the simmering liquid and gently turn fruit with a large spoon. Cook for 5 minutes. Remove from liquid and let cool. Reserve some of the cooking liquid to drizzle over the fruit when serving, if desired.

3. When fruit and liquid have cooled, place in the refrigerator for a couple of hours. Fruit can also be served warm.

4. Serve ½ pear, ½ peach, and ½ plum for each serving. You may slice fruit and fan out on the plate for a lovely presentation. Drizzle a spoonful of the poaching liquid over each serving, if desired.

Variation: Use red wine, which will add a nice pink color to the fruit.

HEALTHY MORSELS

Cinnamon is known for many possible health benefits including anticlotting and antimicrobial properties and regulating blood sugar. Ground cinnamon is an excellent source of manganese and a good source of fiber, vitamin K, calcium, and iron.

Mixed Berry Torte

Sweet berries and creamy, orange-kissed ricotta make a delicious summer treat.

Yield:	Prep time:	Cook time:	Serving size:
12 pieces	30 minutes	15 minutes	1 slice

Each serving has:			
250 calories	11 g total fat	7 g saturated fat	5 g protein
32 g carbohydrates	2 g fiber	30 mg cholesterol	20 mg sodium

⅓ cup granulated sugar

½ cup unsalted butter, softened

2 cups all-purpose flour

4 TB. orange liqueur or orange juice

1 cup ricotta cheese

1 TB. orange zest

1 TB. honey

2 TB. confectioners' sugar

1 pint fresh blueberries, washed and dried

8 oz. fresh strawberries, washed, stemmed, and dried; sliced

Additional confectioners' sugar for garnish

1. Preheat oven to 350°F.

2. Combine sugar, butter, flour, and liqueur in a food processor. Pulse several times or until a dough ball forms. Remove dough and flatten into a disc shape and then press it into a 10-inch tart pan with a removable bottom.

3. Press dough evenly to cover the bottom of the pan. Prick the dough with a fork all over.

4. Bake 15 to 20 minutes or until slightly golden brown. Remove and let cool to room temperature.

5. Combine ricotta cheese, orange zest, honey, and confectioners' sugar. Spread evenly over top of cooled crust.

6. Arrange berries on top of ricotta mixture. Chill for 2 hours and serve. Garnish with confectioners' sugar.

Variation: Use any kind of berries and create a beautiful arrangement.

Berry Sorbet

Sorbet is sweet, refreshing, and very easy to make and goes perfectly with refreshing summer berries.

Yield:	Prep time:	Cook time:	Serving size:
4 cups	10 minutes	30 minutes	½ cup

Each serving has:			
140 calories	0 g total fat	0 g saturated fat	1 g protein
32 g carbohydrates	2 g fiber	0 mg cholesterol	0 mg sodium

2 cups raspberries, washed, dried, and chopped

1 cup strawberries, stemmed, washed, and dried; finely diced

1 cup sugar

2 TB. orange flavored liqueur or orange juice

1. In a large bowl, combine raspberries, strawberries, sugar, orange liqueur, and 1 cup water.

2. Pour mixture into an ice cream maker. Follow the manufacturer's guidelines and let run for 30 minutes or until frozen.

Variation: If you do not own an ice cream maker, you can still make sorbet by freezing it for about 8 hours. You will have to scrape it with a fork several times during the freezing process to prevent it from freezing solid. It will have larger ice crystals, making the texture and consistency different—more similar to an Italian ice.

Fruit and Cheese Plate

Fruit is the perfect accompaniment to cheese and acts as a flavor catalyst. The toasted nuts and the pomegranate seeds are a crunchy and sweet contrast to the savory cheese. This makes a great dessert during the winter or any season.

Yield:	Prep time:	Cook time:	Serving size:
4 servings	15 minutes	None	½ of recipe

Each serving has:			
330 calories	21 g total fat	8 g saturated fat	16 g protein
22 g carbohydrates	4 g fiber	45 mg cholesterol	370 mg sodium

4 Medjool dates	3 oz. manchego cheese
1 oz. walnuts, toasted	3 oz. fontina cheese
1 oz. almonds, toasted	1 TB. honey
1 pear, cored and sliced	¼ cup pomegranate seeds

1. Arrange dates, walnuts, almonds, pear slices, and manchego and fontina cheeses on a platter.

2. Drizzle honey over pear slices and sprinkle with pomegranate seeds.

Variation: Any type of cheese will do instead of fontina. If you don't have fresh fruit on hand, try using a chutney.

HEALTHY MORSELS

Fontina cheese is a classic Italian cheese made from cow's milk. It can be semi-soft to firm in texture, and the flavors can vary depending on where the cheese comes from and how long it has been aged. It can be eaten on its own, used in recipes, or even used as a fondue since it melts well.

Baked Stuffed Peaches

Sweet summer peaches are filled with a mixture of crunchy oats and nuts—like a peach pie without the crust and all the work of a pie!

Yield:	Prep time:	Cook time:	Serving size:
8 servings	10 minutes	15–20 minutes	½ peach
Each serving has:			
175 calories	10 g total fat	5 g saturated fat	3 g protein
20 g carbohydrates	3 g fiber	60 mg cholesterol	65 mg sodium

4 medium fresh peaches, halved
    and pitted

¾ cup rolled oats

½ cup unsweetened coconut

¼ cup chopped pistachios

3 TB. brown sugar

2 egg yolks

½ tsp. vanilla extract

2 TB. butter, at room temperature

1 TB. honey

¼ tsp. kosher salt

1. Preheat oven to 400°F.

2. Scoop out ¼ of the flesh from the center of each peach half and discard to make room for the filling.

3. In a medium bowl, combine oats, coconut, pistachios, brown sugar, egg yolks, vanilla, butter, honey, and salt. Blend well.

4. Divide the oat mixture evenly between peach halves.

5. In a greased ovenproof dish, place peach halves side by side.

6. Bake for 15 to 20 minutes or until oat mixture is golden brown. Serve hot or cold.

Variation: Replace the coconut with the same measurement of any dried fruit such as cranberries, blueberries, or cherries. Substitute almonds or walnuts for the pistachios.

Lemon Ricotta Muffins

Fresh lemon flavor permeates the sweet ricotta cheese and creates the perfect spring muffins.

Yield:	Prep time:	Cook time:	Serving size:
12 muffins	15 minutes	20 minutes	1 muffin

Each serving has:			
260 calories	10 g total fat	6g saturated fat	5 g protein
36 g carbohydrates	5 g fiber	45 mg cholesterol	210 mg sodium

1 cup sugar	Juice and zest of one lemon
½ cup butter, softened	1¾ cups all-purpose flour
½ cup reduced-fat milk	¼ cup cornmeal
1 cup ricotta cheese	2 tsp. baking powder
1 tsp. vanilla extract	½ tsp. kosher salt
1 egg, beaten	Confectioners' sugar for garnish

1. Preheat oven to 350°F.

2. Cream sugar and butter in a mixer for 2 minutes.

3. Add milk, ricotta, vanilla, egg, and lemon juice and zest. Mix on medium speed 1 to 2 minutes or until well combined.

4. In a small bowl, combine flour, cornmeal, baking powder, and salt. Mix well.

5. Add flour mixture to milk mixture and fold gently until just combined.

6. Spray muffin pan with nonstick spray or use paper muffin pan liners. Divide batter to make 12 muffins, about ¼ cup batter each.

7. Bake 20 minutes or until golden brown.

8. Sprinkle with confectioners' sugar, if desired.

Variation: Replace the lemon with any other citrus fruit.

Baklava

Sweet and flaky phyllo dough laced with honey and walnuts is scrumptious in the fall or any season!

Yield:	Prep time:	Cook time:	Serving size:
16 pieces	45 minutes	45–50 minutes	1 piece
Each serving has:			
390 calories	28 g total fat	7 g saturated fat	6 g protein
33 g carbohydrates	2 g fiber	25 mg cholesterol	85 mg sodium

1 lb. walnuts, finely chopped using food processor

¼ cup sugar

1 tsp. ground cinnamon

¼ tsp. ground cloves

14 sheets phyllo dough, thawed according to package directions

1¼ cups butter, melted

1 cup sugar

3 oz. orange blossom honey

1 TB. freshly squeezed lemon juice

1 cinnamon stick

1. Preheat oven to 350°F.

2. Lightly butter bottom and sides of a 9×13 baking pan.

3. In a medium bowl, combine walnuts, sugar, ground cinnamon, and cloves.

4. Lay out one sheet of phyllo dough and brush with melted butter using a pastry brush. Fold phyllo dough in half and place in baking pan.

5. Repeat this process with four more sheets of phyllo dough, working with one sheet at a time.

6. Spread ⅓ nut mixture evenly on top of the layered phyllo dough.

7. Repeat procedure twice more using two layered sheets of phyllo dough at a time, ending with a top layer of nuts.

8. Place five more buttered, folded sheets of phyllo dough on top of nut mixture (repeat step 3 five times).

9. Trim edges of phyllo dough with a sharp knife to make a clean cut around the edges of the pan.

10. Chill pastry for about an hour, allowing the butter to firm up the mixture prior to cutting.

11. Remove pastry from refrigerator. Cut four equal rows down the shortest width of the pan from top to bottom. Cut horizontally down the center or side to create 8 squares. Slice each square diagonally to get 16 triangles.

12. Bake for 45 to 50 minutes or until golden brown.

13. While baklava is baking, combine sugar, ¾ cup water, honey, lemon juice, and cinnamon stick in a small saucepan. Bring to a boil over medium-high heat, then lower the temperature and simmer for 10 minutes. Remove from heat and cool to lukewarm. Discard cinnamon stick.

14. Pour syrup over hot baked baklava. Let stand overnight at room temperature so the syrup is absorbed.

Variation: Add different nuts such as almonds and flavorings such as orange zest to your syrup.

GOOD TO KNOW

Lay out your stack of phyllo dough and pull off one sheet at a time to work with. Lay a damp towel over the stack of phyllo dough to keep it from drying out.

Almond Cookies

Crispy and sweet with a delicate crumb, these cookies are a tasty treat any time of year.

Yield:	Prep time:	Cook time:	Serving size:
30 cookies	20 minutes	15 minutes	1 cookie

Each serving has:			
120 calories	8 g total fat	4 g saturated fat	2 g protein
11 g carbohydrates	1 g fiber	15 mg cholesterol	10 mg sodium

1 cup unsalted butter, softened

½ cup sugar

2 cups all-purpose flour

½ tsp. baking powder

¾ cup raw almonds, finely ground using food processor

1. Preheat oven to 350°F.

2. In a mixing bowl, cream butter and sugar.

3. In a medium bowl, combine flour, baking powder, and almonds. Add to creamed sugar.

4. Mix on low for about 30 seconds. Increase speed and continue mixing for 1 to 2 minutes until well combined.

5. Scoop cookie dough with a tablespoon onto a greased cookie sheet. Chill 1 to 2 hours prior to baking.

6. Bake 15 to 20 minutes or until slightly golden brown.

Variation: Add 1 teaspoon lemon, lime, or orange zest.

Walnut Cake

Light and sweet with a tender crumb, this cake is excellent anytime—and it's especially nice in the winter with a cup of hot coffee.

Yield:	Prep time:	Cook time:	Serving size:
12 pieces	10 minutes	20–25 minutes	1 square

Each serving has:			
200 calories	10 g total fat	1.5 g saturated fat	4 g protein
25 g carbohydrates	1 g fiber	0 mg cholesterol	125 mg sodium

1½ cups all-purpose flour	¼ cup extra-virgin olive oil
½ cup sugar	¾ cup reduced-fat milk
2½ tsp. baking powder	¾ cup walnuts, chopped
¼ tsp. salt	Confectioners' sugar for garnish
1 egg	

1. Position rack in the center of the oven and preheat to 350°F.

2. Lightly grease and flour the bottom of an 8×8 baking pan.

3. In a large bowl, combine flour, sugar, baking powder, and salt.

4. In a medium bowl, beat together egg, oil, and milk.

5. Add egg mixture to flour mixture. Mix until incorporated.

6. Add chopped walnuts into batter, mixing well to combine.

7. Pour batter into the prepared pan. Bake for 20 to 25 minutes or until a toothpick inserted into the center of the cake comes out clean.

8. Remove pan from oven and cool on a wire rack.

9. Transfer to a serving platter and dust with confectioners' sugar. Serve warm or at room temperature.

Variation: Add ½ cup dried cranberries or raisins.

Orange Rice Pudding

The sweet flavor of the orange and cinnamon accents the creamy rice and makes for a wonderful winter-time dessert.

Yield:	Prep time:	Cook time:	Serving size:
3 cups	10 minutes	30 minutes	½ cup

Each serving has:			
190 calories	2 g total fat	1.5 g saturated fat	6 g protein
35 g carbohydrates	2 g fiber	10 mg cholesterol	120 mg sodium

1 cup short-grain white rice

2½ cups reduced-fat milk

1 tsp. vanilla extract

1 tsp. ground cinnamon

¼ tsp. kosher salt

1 large orange

1 TB. orange liqueur or orange juice

1. In a medium saucepan, combine rice, milk, vanilla, cinnamon, and salt. Bring to a boil, then reduce heat to a simmer. Cook for about 15 minutes.

2. While rice is cooking, cut orange into segments with the following method. On a cutting board, cut off top and bottom of orange. Place orange cut side down on the cutting board. Cut off skin and white pith, slicing around orange from top to bottom. Holding orange over a bowl to catch any juices, cut segments out of orange, leaving the membrane between each section behind. Place orange segments in a small bowl. Squeeze juice from the membranes into the rice mixture.

3. When rice has cooked for 15 minutes, stir and cover. Continue cooking for 15 additional minutes or until all liquid has been absorbed.

4. Stir in liqueur and add orange segments.

5. Serve warm or cold.

Variation: Add ½ cup golden raisins and ½ cup toasted coconut.

Fig and Apricot Compote

The sweet and sour spice makes this a great spread for any type of bread or cracker.

Yield:	Prep time:	Cook time:	Serving size:
3 cups	10 minutes	45–60 minutes	¼ cup

Each serving has:			
170 calories	0 g total fat	0 g saturated fat	1 g protein
45 g carbohydrates	3 g fiber	0 mg cholesterol	15 mg sodium

8 oz. dried figs, stems removed	1 cup sugar
6 oz. dried apricots	2 cups water
3 oz. crystallized ginger	1 lemon, juiced
2 cinnamon sticks	1 tsp. apple cider vinegar

1. Place figs in a food processor and pulse until finely chopped. Transfer to a medium saucepan.

2. Place apricots and ginger in food processor and pulse until finely chopped. Do not overload the food processor because fruit is sticky; you want fruit evenly diced. Transfer apricots and ginger to the pan with figs.

3. Add cinnamon sticks, sugar, lemon juice, vinegar, and 2 cups water to pan. Stir to combine ingredients.

4. Bring ingredients to a boil over medium heat. Reduce heat and simmer 45 to 60 minutes, stirring occasionally, until most of the liquid has evaporated.

Variation: Try any type of dried fruit, like cherries, blueberries, or raisins.

Seasonal Menu Plans

In This Chapter

- Best to plan ahead
- Savory summer menus
- Flavorful fall menus
- Warm winter menus
- Lighter spring menus

Now that you have a firm grasp on what foods are included in the Mediterranean diet and why, it is time to put it all together. It you want to stay on track with your new style of Mediterranean eating, your best bet is to plan your menus ahead of time. Planning ahead will ensure that you are prepared, stay on track, always have healthy Mediterranean foods on hand, make fewer trips to the grocery store, and increase the variety of foods you eat each day. Use the Mediterranean Diet Pyramid from Chapter 3 as a guide. Once you plan your menus for the week, you can create your grocery list and make shopping a breeze.

To help you get started, we have created one week of menu plans for each season that incorporate foods of the Mediterranean and many of the recipes found in Part 4. Use the menus as is or make changes so they fit your personal tastes and lifestyle. Before you know it, you will be naturally including all the foods from the Mediterranean diet with ease and incorporating a heart-healthy diet plan into your everyday life. These menus are designed to be convenient. They enable you to have ingredients on hand for the entire week so that you can use them throughout the week in various ways. Chapter 13 will give you ideas for wine pairings if you so desire.

In the following seasonal menus, note that some meals have an asterisk (*) beside the name—this indicates that the recipe is included in this book. The remaining menu items are meal suggestions that you can just whip up yourself. Some of the recipes are used in multiple meal plans, as the growing seasons vary in different regions. Labeling the menu plans by season is only a guide to help you learn to eat a variety of Mediterranean foods throughout the year.

Seven-Day Summer Menu Plan

Summer offers an abundance of fresh fruits and vegetables at their peak flavors. Just because we can purchase almost any fruit and vegetable anytime of the year doesn't mean we should. If a food is in season, it tends to be fresher and last longer. One way to learn what is in season in your area is to visit your local farmers' market. Summer melons, berries, and tomatoes come to mind. A tomato out of season hardly has the same flavor as one just picked off the vine. Summertime is a time when folks dust off their grills and have backyard barbeques. Grill up some extra fish, lean meats, and veggies, which can be used for sandwiches and salads throughout the week.

Day 1

Breakfast: Whole-grain waffle with fresh blueberries and low-fat Greek yogurt

Lunch: *Spinach, Orange, and Feta Salad; *Caramelized Onion Flatbread

Snack: A handful of walnuts and grapes

Dinner: *Pan-Seared Orange Scallops; *Minted Cucumber Salad; steamed zucchini, tomatoes, and onions drizzled with extra-virgin olive oil

Snack: *Tomato Basil Bocconcini

Day 2

Breakfast: Oatmeal with nuts, honey, and fresh raspberries

Lunch: *Gazpacho; *Smoked Salmon Bites

Snack: Strawberries

Dinner: Grilled lamb chops with *Pesto; *Golden Couscous Salad

Snack: *Lemon Minted Melon

Day 3

Breakfast: Scrambled egg wrap with tomatoes, feta, and spinach; fat-free milk

Lunch: Grilled chicken; *Zucchini and Walnuts; couscous; *Classic Mixed Greens Salad with Balsamic Vinaigrette

Snack: Sliced watermelon

Dinner: *Prosciutto and Roasted Vegetable Panini; *Baked Stuffed Peaches

Snack: *Pear, Cheese, and Balsamic Flatbread

Day 4

Breakfast: Low-fat Greek yogurt mixed-berry parfait with granola

Lunch: *Shrimp and Melon Salad

Snack: A handful of almonds and grapes

Dinner: *Hummus; roasted vegetable wrap; *Berry Sorbet

Snack: Strawberries with balsamic reduction

Day 5

Breakfast: Fresh raspberries with melted fontina cheese on toast

Lunch: *Chicken Tzatziki Pita; *Pickled Asparagus

Snack: Fresh cherries and handful of walnuts

Dinner: *Angel Hair Pasta with Pesto, Mushrooms, and Arugula

Snack: *Lemon Ricotta Muffin

Day 6

Breakfast: Blueberry yogurt smoothie

Lunch: *Tomato Basil Pizza; *Poached Summer Fruit with yogurt

Snack: A handful of walnuts

Dinner: *Crab Cakes; *Lemon Kale Ribbons; *Roasted Red Pepper Tapenade

Snack: Sliced watermelon

Day 7

Breakfast: *Baked Vegetable Omelet; fat-free milk

Lunch: *Melon, Prosciutto, and Figs

Snack: Strawberries and almonds

Dinner: Grilled halibut; *Golden Chard; quinoa; *Mixed Berry Torte

Snack: Eggplant dip with celery, carrots, and red bell pepper

Seven-Day Fall Menu Plan

Fall is a transitional time where we have the bounty of leftovers from summer fruits and vegetables that survive until the temperatures drop too low. Fall vegetables like kale and root vegetables are a heartier fare and require a little more preparation. Roasting vegetables helps to draw out and concentrate their flavors.

Day 1

Breakfast: *Baked Vegetable Omelet; fat-free milk

Lunch: *Mushroom, Artichoke, and Arugula Flatbread

Snack: Nectarine

Dinner: Grilled chicken apple sausage; *Barley and Vegetable Sauté; baked acorn squash

Snack: Dried cherries and pecans

Day 2

Breakfast: Oatmeal with cinnamon apples

Lunch: *Chicken Almond Wrap

Snack: Red and green seedless grapes

Dinner: *Split Pea Soup; *Classic Mixed Greens Salad with Balsamic Vinaigrette; *Parmesan Pepper Crisps

Snack: *Stuffed Dates

Day 3

Breakfast: Whole-grain waffle with orange sections and low-fat yogurt

Lunch: *Tuna Salad with Capers and Potatoes

Snack: A handful of almonds and dried apricots

Dinner: *Two-Cheese Risotto; *Cinnamon Apple Nut Phyllo Rolls

Snack: *Hummus with *Parmesan Pepper Crisps

Day 4

Breakfast: Apple cinnamon yogurt smoothie

Lunch: *Mixed Bean Soup; *Mushroom Crostini

Snack: A handful of cashews

Dinner: *Caramelized Onion Flatbread; *Classic Mixed Greens Salad with Balsamic Vinaigrette

Snack: Figs, olives, and mozzarella

Day 5

Breakfast: Scrambled egg wrap with roasted red peppers and onions; fat-free milk

Lunch: *Eggplant Rolls; *Quinoa Pilaf

Snack: Orange

Dinner: *Bean and Vegetable Patties; steamed broccoli; *Baklava

Snack: Olives; crusty bread dipped in extra-virgin olive oil

Day 6

Breakfast: Yogurt parfait with diced pears and blueberries

Lunch: Grilled chicken breast; patty pan squash sautéed with garlic; *Tabbouleh Salad

Snack: Apple

Dinner: *Fish Stew; crusty bread; *Classic Mixed Greens Salad with Balsamic Vinaigrette

Snack: Toasted almonds and pomegranate seeds

Day 7

Breakfast: *Pear, Cheese, and Balsamic Flatbread

Lunch: *Roasted Beet Salad; *Onion Apple Marmalade on crusty bread

Snack: Orange

Dinner: *Lamb Shanks; garlic mashed potatoes; sautéed spinach

Snack: Eggplant dip with whole-wheat pita wedges

Seven-Day Winter Menu Plan

Cold winter days are a good time to make use of kitchen staples. A well-stocked pantry can help you whip up a delicious meal regardless of the weather outside. Take advantage of cooking dried beans and pastas with canned ingredients like artichoke hearts, tomatoes, and corn. Dried ingredients like raisins, sun-dried tomatoes, figs, and dates are also wonderful to use in winter. Focus on hot foods to warm you from the inside out!

Day 1

Breakfast: Poached egg on toast; blood orange sections; fat-free milk

Lunch: *Lemon Lentil Soup; *Parmesan Pepper Crisps; *Classic Mixed Greens Salad with Balsamic Vinaigrette

Snack: Low-fat Greek yogurt; almonds; apple wedges

Dinner: Roasted chicken; *Rosemary Garlic Potatoes; broccoli rabe

Snack: *Orange Rice Pudding

Day 2

Breakfast: Yogurt parfait with diced pear

Lunch: *Marinated Artichoke Salad; ½ turkey sandwich

Snack: Dried fruit and walnuts

Dinner: *Salmon Fennel Bundles; couscous; baby carrots

Snack: *Lemon Ricotta Muffin

Day 3

Breakfast: Oatmeal with toasted almonds and orange segments; fat-free milk

Lunch: *Tomato Basil Soup; *Classic Mixed Greens Salad with Balsamic Vinaigrette

Snack: Low-fat yogurt and apple wedges

Dinner: *Lamb Patties (without pasta); *Sweet Polenta with Sun-Dried Tomatoes; roasted Brussels sprouts

Snack: Olive tapenade on toasted baguette slice

Day 4

Breakfast: Tangerine segments and melted Fontina cheese on toast

Lunch: *Fennel and Apple Salad; roasted chicken

Snack: Cashews; low-fat mozzarella cheese; olives

Dinner: *Crispy Turkey Cutlets; *Curried Cauliflower; red kidney beans

Snack: *Walnut Cake

Day 5

Breakfast: Oatmeal with almonds, pears, and honey

Lunch: *Caramelized Onion Flatbread; spaghetti squash with chickpeas and feta

Snack: Orange sections drizzled with extra-virgin olive oil

Dinner: *Butternut Squash Soup; ½ cheese panini; *Classic Mixed Greens Salad with Balsamic Vinaigrette

Snack: Olives; crusty bread dipped in extra-virgin olive oil

Day 6

Breakfast: Whole-grain waffle with sliced apples; low-fat yogurt

Lunch: Tuna salad wrap with avocado slices

Snack: Pear

Dinner: *Spicy Tomato Sauce with Linguine; chicken apple sausage; sautéed zucchini

Snack: *Stuffed Dates

Day 7

Breakfast: *Baked Vegetable Omelet; blood orange sections; fat-free milk

Lunch: Turkey panini; watercress salad; cup of minestrone soup

Snack: Low-fat Greek yogurt and walnuts

Dinner: *Butternut Squash and Goat Cheese Pizza

Snack: *Fig and Apricot Compote; *Onion Apple Marmalade on crusty bread

Seven-Day Spring Menu Plan

Spring emerges with delicate leafy greens, asparagus, and artichokes. You can even plant your own leafy greens. You just need to protect them from a late frost by covering them if the temperature dips low. These spring menus are lighter but still satisfying.

Day 1

Breakfast: *Baked Vegetable Omelet; fat-free milk

Lunch: *Prosciutto and Roasted Vegetable Panini; avocado slices

Snack: Low-fat Greek yogurt and kumquats

Dinner: *Chicken Piccata; *Sautéed Spinach and Mushrooms; white kidney beans; *Vanilla Panna Cotta

Snack: Tangelo and a handful of pecans

Day 2

Breakfast: Low-fat Greek yogurt parfait with apple and granola

Lunch: *Vegetable Orzo Soup; ½ turkey sandwich

Snack: Dried apricots and a handful of walnuts

Dinner: *Sole Florentine; *Rosemary Garlic Potatoes; roasted peppers; *Almond Cookies

Snack: *Hummus with celery and carrot sticks

Day 3

Breakfast: Oatmeal with walnuts and honey

Lunch: *Chicken Almond Wrap; steamed asparagus

Snack: Low-fat yogurt and apple wedges

Dinner: *Panzanella with turkey; *Orange Rice Pudding

Snack: *Fruit and Cheese Plate

Day 4

Breakfast: Frozen blueberry yogurt smoothie

Lunch: *Tuna Salad with Capers and Potatoes

Snack: Blood orange segments drizzled with extra-virgin olive oil and chopped pistachios

Dinner: Appetizer quartet: *Lamb Pesto Crostini; *Roasted Red Pepper Tapenade; *Onion Apple Marmalade; *Pickled Asparagus

Snack: *Hummus with carrots, radishes, and celery sticks

Day 5

Breakfast: Scrambled egg wrap with feta, mushrooms, and spinach; tangerine segments; fat-free milk

Lunch: *Lemon Lentil Soup; ½ cheese panini

Snack: Cashews; dried cherries and blueberries

Dinner: *Spicy Tomato Sauce with Linguine; *Classic Mixed Greens Salad with Balsamic Vinaigrette

Snack: Olives; crusty bread dipped in extra-virgin olive oil

Day 6

Breakfast: Whole-grain waffle with apple slices and low-fat yogurt

Lunch: *Mushroom, Artichoke, and Arugula Flatbread

Snack: Dried dates and apricots with walnuts

Dinner: *Almond-Crusted Barramundi; *Minted Peas with Pancetta; quinoa; *Almond Cookies

Snack: *Roasted Red Pepper Tapenade with whole-wheat pita bread

Day 7

Breakfast: Broiled pink grapefruit with brown sugar and low-fat Greek yogurt

Lunch: *Spinach, Orange, and Feta Salad; cup of vegetable soup

Snack: Apple wedges with manchego cheese

Dinner: *Lamb Patties and Pasta; *Classic Mixed Greens Salad with Balsamic Vinaigrette

Snack: *Lemon Cannellini Spread with toasted whole-wheat flatbread

Glossary

alpha linolenic acid (ALA)   Omega-3 fatty acids found in plant sources.

amino acids   The building blocks that make up protein.

antioxidants   A group of nutrients that counteract effects of harmful free radicals.

body mass index   An index calculated using height and weight to determine a person's healthy weight range.

capers   Immature buds plucked from a small bush that is native to the Mediterranean and Middle East.

carbohydrates   An organic compound consisting of carbon, hydrogen, and oxygen. A component of food that provides calories and energy to the body.

cardiovascular disease   A class of diseases that involve the heart and/or the blood vessels including the arteries and veins.

cholesterol   A soft waxy substance that is found among the lipids or fats in the bloodstream and in the cells of the body. Dietary cholesterol is found in animal foods.

complete protein   A protein that provides the body with an adequate proportion of all nine essential amino acids needed for optimal health.

complex carbohydrates (starches)   Three or more simple sugars that are linked together. Also called *polysaccharides*.

coronary artery disease   *See* coronary heart disease (CHD).

coronary heart disease (CHD)   A narrowing of the small blood vessels that supply both blood and oxygen to the heart.

DASH Diet   Stands for "Dietary Approaches to Stop Hypertension." A heart-healthy diet to help people manage their high blood pressure.

diabetes   Refers to a group of diseases that are evident by high levels of blood glucose or blood sugar due to defects in either the production or action of insulin (a hormone in the body) or both.

Dietary Guidelines for Americans   Science- and evidence-based nutritional and fitness goals that promote health and are meant to help reduce the risk of chronic disease.

Dietary Reference Intakes (DRI)   Daily nutrient recommendations for Americans based on age and gender that are set by the Institute of Medicine's Food and Nutrition Board (FNB). Expressed as RDA (recommended daily allowance) or AI (adequate intake).

disaccharides   *See* simple carbohydrates.

diverticulosis   A condition of the colon in which tiny pouches or diverticula form on the colon walls. When these pouches become infected or inflamed, the condition is known as diverticulitis.

docosahexaenoic acid (DHA)   An omega-3 fatty acid exclusively found in fish and seafood.

eicosapentaenoic acid (EPA)   An omega-3 fatty acid exclusively found in fish and seafood.

empty calorie foods   Foods that are high in calories but low in nutritional content.

enriched   When nutrients are added back to a food that were removed in processing.

fat-soluble vitamins   Vitamins that dissolve in fat and are carried through the bloodstream and the body through fat (vitamins A, D, E, and K).

free radicals   Highly reactive atoms or groups of atoms with an unpaired electron; they can come from the environment such as cigarette smoke, pollution, and ultraviolet light. Free radicals are also the by-product of the body using oxygen. Free radicals cause damage to body cells.

fructose   The natural sugar found in fruit.

glucose   A simple sugar found in some foods that the body uses as a source of energy. It also circulates in the blood as blood glucose or blood sugar.

gluten   A mixture of proteins found in wheat, rye, barley, and other foods. It's what gives bread the elasticity and structure that allows it to rise.

glycemic index (GI)   A numerical scale that indicates how fast a single food raises blood glucose (blood sugar).

healthy fats   Fats that are unsaturated such as monounsaturated, polyunsaturated, and omega-3 fatty acids. These fats help to reduce the risk for heart disease.

heme iron   The form of most iron found in animal foods.

high-density lipoproteins (HDL)   Referred to as "good" cholesterol. Rids the body of dietary cholesterol, which lowers your risk for heart disease.

hydrogenation   The process by which liquid vegetable oil is made more solid by the addition of hydrogen.

hypertension   The medical term used for high blood pressure.

incomplete protein   A protein that does not include all nine essential amino acids or does not include all nine in adequate amounts. Found in most plant proteins.

insoluble fiber   A type of fiber found in plants that the body cannot digest and does not break down as it passes through the digestive tract. Helps to promote regularity.

ketogenic diet   Diets that severely restrict carbohydrates and are high in protein and fat. These diets trigger short-term weight loss. *See also* ketosis.

ketosis   Abnormal accumulation of ketones in the body that occurs when the diet lacks enough carbohydrates, the body's main source of energy, and results in an excessive breakdown of fats.

lactose   The natural sugar found in dairy products such as milk.

lavash   Flatbread of Middle Eastern origin.

legumes   A category of plants that have pods (or fruits) and include beans, peas, lentils, and peanuts.

lipids   A general term that refers to all fats, cholesterol, and fatlike substances.

low-density lipoproteins (LDL)   Referred to as "bad" cholesterol. Causes cholesterol buildup in artery walls, which increases the risk for heart disease and stroke.

Mediterranean Diet Pyramid   Visually represents the most current nutritional research that represents a healthy, traditional Mediterranean diet.

metabolism   The process by which the body uses or burns calories for energy.

micronutrients   *See* vitamins; minerals.

minerals Inorganic compounds essential to the body for various functions. Minerals come in two categories: major and trace. Major minerals are needed by the body in greater amounts than trace minerals.

monosaccharides *See* simple carbohydrates.

monounsaturated fats (MUFA) Fats that are missing one hydrogen pair on their chemical chain. They are typically liquid at room temperature but will solidify when chilled. Considered a heart-healthy fat.

nonheme iron The type of most iron found in plant foods.

nutrient-dense foods Foods that contain vitamins, minerals, fiber, and other essential nutrients yet are low in calories.

Nutrition Facts Panel The box on food labels that provide required nutritional information.

omega-3 fatty acids A group of essential polyunsaturated fatty acids that are considered heart healthy and health-promoting. Our body cannot produce them, so we must get them from the foods we eat.

omega-6 fatty acids A group of essential polyunsaturated fatty acids. Although they are essential, the amount we should consume has been controversial.

orzo Small, rice-shaped pasta.

pancetta A pork product that is similar to bacon except pancetta is not smoked.

phytochemicals *See* phytonutrients.

phytonutrients Naturally occurring compounds found in plant-based foods that offer potential health benefits.

plant sterols/stanols Substances found naturally in fruits, vegetables, and plant oils that have been found to lower LDL cholesterol.

polysaccharides *See* complex carbohydrates.

polyunsaturated fats Fats that have more than one missing hydrogen pair on their chemical chain. These fats are typically liquid at room temperature and when chilled. Considered a healthy fat.

probiotics Live microorganisms (usually bacteria) that are similar to beneficial microorganisms found in our gut. They are good bacteria that may treat and prevent certain illnesses and support general health. An example is the live bacterial cultures found in yogurt.

proteins   A macronutrient that is found both in the foods that we eat and in many structures of the body.

refined grains   Whole grains that have been processed or milled and have had the bran and germ removed.

saturated fats   Fats with a chemical structure that is saturated with hydrogen. They are solid at room temperature and can increase total and bad cholesterol, raising one's risk for heart disease, stroke, and cancer.

simple carbohydrates (simple sugars)   Single sugar units or pairs of sugar units linked together.

soluble fiber   A type of fiber in plant foods that dissolves easily in water and takes on a soft, gel-like form in the intestines. Helps lower cholesterol and regulate blood sugar.

smoke point   The temperature at which the oil will smoke when heated.

trans fats   Fats that raise total and bad cholesterol, lower good cholesterol, and increase the risk for heart disease and stroke. Produced when liquid fats are put through the hydrogenation process.

triglycerides   The main form of fat in foods. Excess calories from any type of food source are processed in the body and changed to triglycerides for storage as fat in the body.

vitamins   Organic compounds and a group of nutrients that are required in small amounts for optimal health.

water-soluble vitamins   Vitamins that dissolve in water and are carried through the body by watery fluids (eight B vitamins plus vitamin C).

whole grains   Grains that are made up of the entire seed of the grain, containing the three key parts: bran, germ, and endosperm.

Online Resources

The following online resources will help to further your knowledge, keep you up to date with new findings, and open the door to discovering more about the Mediterranean diet and good health. This information was reliable and correct at the time of this writing; we assume no responsibility for any recent changes in contact information that may have occurred since the initial printing of this book.

Websites

American Cancer Society   www.cancer.org

American Diabetes Association   www.diabetes.org

American Dietetic Association   www.eatright.org

American Heart Association   www.heart.org

American Institute for Cancer Research   www.aicr.org

Consumerlab.com   www.consumerlab.com

Farmers' Market Directory   www.ams.usda.gov/AMSv1.0/FarmersMarkets

Fats of Life   www.fatsoflife.com

Mediterranean Diet   www.mediterraneandiet.com

Mediterranean Foods Alliance   mediterraneanmark.org

Nutrition Focus   www.nutrifocus.net

Oldways Preservation & Exchange Trust   www.oldwayspt.org/mediterraneandiet

The Olive Oil Source   www.oliveoilsource.com

Produce for Better Health Foundation   www.pbhfoundation.org

Tufts University Diet and Nutrition Letter   www.healthletter.tufts.edu

USDA Dietary Guidelines for Americans   fnic.nal.usda.gov

USDA's MyPyramid   www.mypyramid.gov

USDA Nutrition.gov   www.nutrition.gov

The Vegetarian Resource Group   www.vrg.org

Whole Grains Council   wholegrainscouncil.org

Women's Heart Foundation   www.womensheart.org

Index